Specific Dyslexia

Specific Dyslexia

The Research Report of the ICAA Word Blind Centre for Dyslexic Children

Sandhya Naidoo MA

Introduction by **Alfred White Franklin**

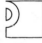

Pitman Publishing

First published 1972

Sir Isaac Pitman and Sons Ltd
Pitman House, Parker Street, Kingsway, London WC2B 5PB
PO Box 46038, Portal Street, Nairobi, Kenya

Sir Isaac Pitman (Aust) Pty Ltd
Pitman House, 158 Bouverie Street, Carlton, Victoria 3053, Australia

Pitman Publishing Company SA Ltd
PO Box 11231, Johannesburg, South Africa

Pitman Publishing Corporation
6 East 43rd Street, New York, NY 10017, USA

Sir Isaac Pitman (Canada) Ltd
495 Wellington Street West, Toronto 135, Canada

The Copp Clark Publishing Company
517 Wellington Street West, Toronto 135, Canada

ISBN: 0 273 36093 0

Printed by photo-lithography and made in Great Britain at the Pitman Press, Bath
G2 (G4647)

Foreword

It gives me much pleasure to express the thanks of the Association to all who made this research possible and to those who carried it through and helped in the preparation of the report. In particular, our thanks go to Dr White Franklin, Mrs Sandhya Naidoo and the professional advisers on the Word Blind Committee.

Dr White Franklin, then Chairman of the ICAA, gave the impetus to the Association to extend its work in this field. Later, as Chairman of the Word Blind Centre's Committee and Honorary Medical Adviser at the Centre, he readily gave of his time and also invaluable practical help in the final preparation of the report. Under his guidance, the members of the Word Blind Committee gave freely of their valuable time and advice. They are listed on page vii and we thank them most warmly for their help

Sir George Haynes, my immediate predecessor, gave his wise advice and support to the project during his time as Chairman of the Association and beyond.

Mrs Naidoo has devoted all her time over the past four years to the direction of the Centre and the research. Her dedicated application has been remarkable, and she has been supported energetically by her colleagues at the Centre and at ICAA central office

The research would not have been possible but for the considerable financial help received from the Children's Research Fund who grant-aided us to the extent of £25,000 over a seven-year period. To them, to the City Parochial Foundation who made a grant of £10,000 over five years, and to the individual donors, we express our warmest thanks.

We are greatly indebted to the Dean and the Institute of Child Health for giving us the use of the premises at Coram's Fields. The Coram's Fields Foundation granted us the use of their facilities and generally played the part of a good neighbour and we express our thanks for their kindness.

Rupert Nevill
Chairman

Word Blind Committee Members

Acknowledgements

It is impossible to thank by name all who contributed directly or indirectly to the research reported here. The writer is grateful to the members of the Word Blind Centre's Committee for their suggestions and advice during the planning and course of this project.

The medical examinations were carried out by Dr A. White Franklin and by Dr Macdonald Critchley, Consulting Physician to the National Hospital for Nervous Diseases, London. With the kind co-operation of Mr Alan Fuller, Consulting Otologist and Dr Geoffery Udall, Senior Lecturer in Child Health, the audiological examinations were made at Saint Bartholomew's Hospital, London. The Centre's Educational Psychologists, Mrs Eileen Ashton, Mrs Sylvia Cohen, Miss Judy Goyen, Mr David Moseley and Mrs Carole Strahan were, with the writer, responsible for the psychological testing, assistance being given by Miss Carole Flesch and Miss Jean Wilson and the Centre's first Research Assistant Mrs Gillian Crewdson. Mrs Crewdson and her successors Mrs Donna Hecks and Mrs Judith Duchemin, with Mr Robert Ford, selected the subjects, prepared the record forms and coded, tabulated and checked the data. Mr Harvey Goldstein, Lecturer in Statistics at the Institute of Child Health, London, advised and helped in computing the statistics and Mr Gavin Ross, of the Statistics Department of the Rothamsted Experimental Station, processed the data for the cluster analysis. Both are warmly thanked. We are indebted to the Inner London Education Authority for their assistance in finding and permitting us to use two schools in their area. Much gratitude is extended to the Head Teachers of these two schools, Mr W. M. Lloyd and Mr M. K. Ross, and to the Heads of the two Independent schools, Mr R. Cooper of The Hall Preparatory School and Mr and Mrs A. N. Ingham of Eaton House School for their co-operation in expediting the selection and examination of the control boys. Parents of dyslexic and control boys are thanked for their painstaking efforts to provide the requested information. Miss Catherine Renfrew, chief Speech Therapist at the Churchill Hospital, Oxford, kindly gave permission to use her Test of Articulation and her advice on scoring it is much appreciated. Thanks are due to the University of London Press Limited for permission to reproduce Form BG1 of the Bristol Social Adjustment Guide.

The original typescript was read by Professor T. R. Miles, Professor of

Psychology, University of Bangor, and the writer is very grateful for his constructive comments and encouragement. The final draft was discussed with Professor O. L. Zangwill, Professor of Psychology, University of Cambridge, whose unfailing support and advice are deeply appreciated. Dr Franklin gave unstintingly of his time and good counsel at each stage in the planning, execution and writing of this work. His invaluable assistance in the preparation of this report is much appreciated and gratefully acknowledged. This work could not have been completed without the constant support of my colleagues at the Word Blind Centre. The ICAA is warmly thanked for being so unfailingly supportive throughout my tenure of office at the Centre. I am particularly grateful to Miss Eileen Hilton, the ICAA's General Secretary.

Finally, I must thank Miss Gwen Heath and Mrs Dorothy Boardman who typed the manuscript and my family who bore patiently and indulgently with my absorption in this report.

S. Naidoo

Contents

Introduction

By Alfred White Franklin

The Invalid Children's Aid Association first concerned itself with the problem of intelligent children with learning difficulties ten years ago, when a panel of experts was invited to talk about "word-blindness" at an Association Council meeting. In April 1962 the Association convened a Conference on Word-blindness or Specific Developmental Dyslexia, addressed by authorities from many countries, and attended by professional people and some parents. A resolution was passed recommending the formation of a "can't read/can't spell parents' association," and copies of the published Proceedings were presented to every Local Education Authority. ICAA felt that while theoretical arguments abounded as to whether or not a special condition of "word-blindness" existed, too little of practical value was being done for the unfortunate children, and that this was largely because basic knowledge was inadequate. The Association therefore decided to seek means for setting up a centre where children, who found learning to read especially difficult, could be referred for a full assessment. When geographically possible, some would be given individual remedial tuition. ICAA felt too that more research was needed, and hoped that fruitful action would follow an end to the arguments. Despite a vast literature, teaching methods remained empirical or followed theories which lacked controlled scientific supporting data.

The ICAA argument was that if a specific condition existed, distinct from the general run of "learning to read" problems, signs and symptoms forming one or more clinically diagnosable syndromes ought to be identifiable. What might be described as profiles of the disorder could then be drawn on which a reliable estimate of prevalence could be based. The effectiveness of the different teaching techniques could be compared and a strong case made for the inclusion within the educational system of remedial tuition, suited to the child's particular difficulties.

While the necessary funds to set up such a centre were being sought, Miss Maisie Holt offered to test one or two children a week at St Bartholomew's Hospital, EC1, medical examinations being carried out in the Department of Child Health. Miss Holt generously placed her considerable experience at the service of the new venture, which owes much to her enthusiasm and drive.

In 1963 the ICAA set up the Word Blind Committee to plan and guide the work. Professional experts were needed, and from the beginning Dr Macdonald

Critchley, Miss Maisie Holt, Professor Patrick Meredith, Professor T. R. Miles and Professor O. L. Zangwill were active members giving generously of their wisdom and their time, as did Dr Kellmer Pringle and Sir Wilfrid Sheldon when later they joined the Committee.

Lack of money and inadequate accommodation delayed matters, but on receipt of the first donation of £2,000 from the late Mrs Arnold Stuart, and as something of an act of faith, an educational psychologist, Dr A. D. Bannatyne, was appointed in April 1964 to conduct the research, working at first at the Association's headquarters in Palace Gate. He set about abstracting all the relevant literature on dyslexia, toured the United States and Denmark, and drew up research proposals which were published in 1965 in *The Word Blind Bulletin*, a periodic publication begun in February 1963.

Both the Children's Research Fund and the City Parochial Foundation had by now agreed to support the project financially and in 1965 the interest and goodwill of Mr Gordon Piller, then House Governor of The Hospital for Sick Children, Great Ormond Street, secured for ICAA a small school building on the point of being demolished in Coram's Fields, on loan from the Institute of Child Health.

The start of the research proper had been delayed because of the difficulty in deciding on a consistent and reliably standardized battery of tests. Meanwhile, once the Centre's existence became known, a steady stream of children began to arrive, and soon school teachers and psychologists were asking to visit and to learn what was happening. With the increased work Mr David Moseley was appointed Research Assistant.

In the summer of 1966 Dr Bannatyne resigned to take up a post in the United States, and the ICAA fortunately acquired the services in September 1966 of another educational psychologist, Mrs Sandhya Naidoo, to direct the research. She was soon invited to become Director of the Centre. Her first task was to reshape the research proposal and then to establish an acceptable battery of tests. The success of her efforts can be seen in the Report here published where her objectives and findings are defined with such clarity.

Apart from research much else was happening at the Centre. Some boys were being taught individually for one or two hours weekly, while continuing general education at school. The biographical material collected illustrates what happens to affected children under present conditions. The emotional reactions and the attitudes of parents, teachers and the children themselves are seen to improve following correct diagnosis and a proper understanding of the true nature of the child's learning difficulties. Progress with remedial reading in clinics and at schools can be compared with the effect of specialized teaching, and the disadvantage of travelling to the Centre balanced against the limitations of school remedial classes. To those with reading problems not fulfilling the criteria laid down for acceptance for assessment, advice was given through Miss Rackham at ICAA Central Office. The large size of this load shows the need for a Central Advisory body to direct at least some of the puzzled parents to existing solutions.

Examining Boards have been persuaded to make some allowance for dyslexic candidates by discarding the idea that slow and poor writing with bad spelling mean illiteracy which is equated with stupidity. A dyslexic candidate writes less and less fully than his non-dyslexic colleagues, but what matters is whether his knowledge of the subject is accurate.

There is still no general agreement that specific dyslexia is a condition differing sufficiently from other kinds of difficulty in reading to require specialized teaching. The 1962 Conference Report and the Word Blind Bulletin have had some effect. So has the formation of Parents' Groups in various parts of the country, who are able to press Local Education Authorities on a case basis. The Colleges of Education plan to pay greater attention to the teaching of reading and some of the difficulties likely to be encountered. School-teachers above all people should be aware of what may go wrong and that they recognize this need is shown by the numbers applying to attend the Centre's special courses in 1969 and 1970. The lectures, with helpful suggestions about teaching, have been published.[1]

This introduction has told briefly the story of the Word Blind Centre for Dyslexic Children, of how ICAA became interested and what it has tried to do for the children and their families. It will be seen that Mrs Naidoo's work has been solidly based and has added a body of valuable knowledge to a subject where exact knowledge has, perhaps, been too little in amount and too little regarded. It has been said that this cool study in an area where great emotion is generated has "taken the heat out of the word-blindness controversies." The ICAA hopes that the publication of the report will substitute a little new light, and with this publication ends the story of the ICAA Word Blind Centre for Dyslexic Children.

The Centre has closed and the staff dispersed. Happily plans for further help have been made for most of the children. Those who have taken part in this enterprise may be allowed to combine with gratitude for the opportunity to serve, a modicum of pride in having gained more recognition and secured more sympathy and help for a group of disadvantaged pupils. They all share disappointment that the day has not yet dawned when responsibility for providing for the special needs of this group is fully recognized throughout the education service. They must be content with the thought that they have brought that dawn a little nearer.

The psychologists, the teachers, the administrative and secretarial staff at the Centre and at headquarters have certainly earned the gratitude of dyslexic children and their families. Many people have contributed much to this project, but special mention must be made of Miss Elizabeth Kirkwood, who as Administrative Secretary bore the burden of organization in the early days, and of Miss Kate Rackham, who gave invaluable help throughout the whole period. The final word is that the research could not have been carried out, nor indeed could any of the Centre's work, without wholehearted support, which includes money along with moral support and trust, from all associated with The Invalid Children's Aid Association.

---

[1] *The Assessment and Teaching of Dyslexic Children,* obtainable from ICAA, 126 Buckingham Palace Road, London, SW1. (Price £1.25.)

1

The Problem—Some Children whose Difficulties are Investigated

This volume is concerned with only a minority of the large total of backward readers. Their disorder, called here specific dyslexia, was identified more than seventy years ago, but only in recent years is its existence being slowly acknowledged. It was first called "congenital word blindness."

The difficulties of dyslexic children are severe and are increased by both lack of recognition and inadequate facilities for diagnosis and teaching. Educational theory and practice have moved far from the era when children went to school primarily to learn the three Rs. But practice is still such that unless the child, and particularly the intelligent child, can learn two of those Rs, Reading and Writing, with some ease, he has little chance of receiving an education commensurate with age, ability and aptitude. Handicapped educationally, he is then too often denied the teaching he needs to develop his potential to the full. Conscious of his failure to succeed as the majority of those around him are succeeding, perhaps under pressure at home as well as at school, he is particularly vulnerable to emotional stresses and strains. When he leaves school his choice of a career may be restricted because of the limitations imposed by his handicap.

Much progress has been made towards an understanding of the difficulties of most retarded readers and towards the provision of help. But for the child with a specific dyslexia facilities for assessment and tuition still lag far behind requirements.

There are many reasons for this tardiness of recognition and lack of provision, not the least of them being the belief that the disorder is a manifestation of emotional disturbance. The multiplicity of terms used to describe reading disorders has added to the confusion. Unfortunately for ease of recognition, dyslexic children do not present clear-cut consistent clinical patterns and many of the features are found in normal readers. But, as Money (1962) has written, "It is not at all rare in psychological medicine, nor in other branches of medicine, that a disease should have no unique identifying sign, that uniqueness being in the pattern of signs that appear in contiguity. Out of context, each sign might also be encountered in other diseases, or, in different intensities, in the healthy. Specific dyslexia is no exception in this respect."

The Word Blind Centre for Dyslexic Children was established by the Invalid Children's Aid Association in 1963, not only to provide facilities for

1

the assessment and teaching of dyslexic children but also to investigate the nature of their difficulties. The workers at the Centre have kept open minds about the reality of specific dyslexia, taking the view that if there be children with a reading disorder which requires facilities for investigation and treatment not normally provided, then it should be possible to produce evidence of the characteristics by which they may be recognized. An accurate diagnosis should be possible. This report of an investigation into the nature and causes of specific dyslexia may best be introduced with a description of a few children who illustrate the problem.

Peter

Peter was 10 years old when he came to the Centre for examination. He could neither read nor write. He could not write his own name, and even made errors when copying it. His difficulties had been noted at his infant school. Since no progress at all had been made in reading by the time he left the infant school, he was seen by the educational psychologist. He was then treated as a slow-learning child and placed in a special class, where he was given a great deal of help, much of it individual. His teacher was both kind and sympathetic. She tried many reading schemes including the Initial Teaching Alphabet, but to no avail. It was clear that Peter was not dull, and his teachers fully agreed with the educational psychologist who had found him to be of average verbal and good average non-verbal intelligence. Peter was a happy, friendly and polite boy and got on well with adults and children. But in the few months before he was seen at the Centre, he was becoming boisterous and difficult to manage. Peter had become very sensitive about his complete failure to read and although he was still responding positively to encouragement, he would avoid anything to do with reading and writing if he possibly could.

His parents were kind, warm-hearted and always supportive. Peter, the youngest of a large family, was regarded as the baby. But he was in no way a "spoiled" child. The family was an ordinary, hard-working and united one. His parents did not expect great academic achievement but they, as well as everyone officially concerned with Peter, were now most troubled about his inability to read. Mother was aware that Peter had been very dependent on her and that this had made it difficult for him to settle into school. She thought at first that this was why Peter did not learn to read, a view shared by the educational psychologist who put the problem down to an emotional block. There had been a further complicating factor. Towards the end of Peter's first year at school, when he had settled in nicely, he was involved in a car accident, sustaining a fractured arm and linear fractures of both parietal skull bones. He had not lost consciousness. He was kept in hospital for just over two weeks and under observation for some time afterwards. No complications developed, recovery was steady and Peter was discharged fit and well after three months.

Mother could not recall whether Peter had begun to read before the accident, but the very full report from the school suggested that he had not.

Peter's history was otherwise uneventful. Mother had developed thrombosis in pregnancy. The baby was, according to mother, two weeks overdue. There were no perinatal or neonatal problems and the baby thrived. He walked and talked at normal ages. But his parents noted, and the examination confirmed, that although articulation was clear, Peter consistently mispronounced certain sounds. Behaviour was never a problem. Apart from the accident his only illnesses had been mumps and measles.

Peter was a healthy, well-grown lad. Vision and hearing were good. The physician's examination elicited no physical or neurological defects and no clumsiness or inco-ordination.

The psychological examination revealed much of interest. Peter had difficulty in discriminating between some sounds which included "th" and "f," "th" and "v," "m" and "n" and he was uncertain about "b" and "g". In speech he invariably used "f" or "v" for "th," sometimes "v" for "b." This created a real problem later for Peter never learned when to write "th" or "f" and would often write "v" for "b." His ability to remember a sequence of digits was very poor. He could recall only a limited number of digits and confused their order. His ability to blend a series of sounds into meaningful words was very poor and some of his errors reflected a serial ordering problem, such as giving "sip" for "c-r-i-s-p."

There was no great difference between verbal and non-verbal ability on the intelligence test, but Peter had considerable difficulty in constructing a pattern from a number of blocks because of his uncertainty about the way the blocks should be turned in order to match the pattern before him. Reversals in reading or writing were not found at the time of examination for the simple reason that Peter could not read and knew few letters to write, but they became very evident as he learned to read and write.

Peter had very confused notions of right and left, the confusion being partly a verbal labelling one. The identification of right and left in relation to his own body was unreliable and he had not yet learned how to identify right and left in people or objects facing him.

He had considerable difficulty on a test of finger localization. He could not repeat the days of the week nor the months of the year.

Peter wrote with the left hand, could throw equally well with either hand but preferred to use the right. He dealt cards with the right hand. He was right-eyed and right-footed.

Father and one of his sisters were left-handed. The family were all good readers but one of his brothers had spelling difficulties.

Until he was asked to read, Peter related excellently to the examiner. He was cheerful, revealed a sense of humour, and enjoyed the varied tasks. He tried hard and concentrated well. When finally it came to reading his manner changed abruptly. He became quiet and tense. He fidgeted and blushed. His hands became so sweaty that he had to wipe them before he could hold a pencil.

Could this really be regarded as a case of reading retardation following an emotional block? We thought not. The deficits elicited on examination were not simply related to reading and were too suggestive of a neurological abnormality. How much resulted from the car accident it is impossible to say in the absence of information about his previous condition. The speech defect had certainly been present before and so had his left-handedness.

Peter's story could be repeated many times with different names and differing details. Peter was fortunate in being well supported both at home and at school. Yet, in spite of this, behavioural problems were beginning to develop and he was afraid to tackle any new task in case it involved reading. He was beginning to withdraw from many activities at school. He was

fortunate, too, in that the local authority was prepared to take further steps
in the identification and treatment of the real problem. But at least two years
had been lost and problems were emerging which might have been prevented.

Martin

When Martin's parents first contacted the Centre, they were almost apologetic.
Their 10-year-old son's problem seemed to be so slight that they wondered if
they ought to be bothering us with it. Martin, they said, could now read quite
fluently but he had had some difficulty in learning to read. Now the difficulty
was getting things down on paper and this was becoming a problem at school.
They had not wished to take any steps to investigate his difficulties before
for fear of creating further problems, but it seemed that Martin was a very
bright boy and they were now afraid that his very poor spelling might become
an educational handicap. Could we help? They wanted to know if there was
anything to be concerned about, and if so, what was the best course of action.

Both parents were highly educated. There were two boys in the family,
Martin being the younger. The elder brother was achieving distinction at
school but father thought that Martin was perhaps, the more highly intelligent.
He had a quick wit but lacked the determination of the older boy. There
seemed to be a very warm relationship between the boys and there was no
trace of any of the resentment Martin might have felt when he compared his
brother's success with his own mediocre achievements at school. The family
presented as an affectionate united one.

On examination, Martin was found to be highly intelligent. His performance
on the verbal intelligence test placed him at the 99th percentile. Although on
the non-verbal part of the intelligence test he scored at a superior level, there
was a significant discrepancy between verbal and non-verbal ability. While
achieving maximum scores on some tests, his scores on reproducing a series
of digits was below average. He could remember the digits but the sequence
was wrong. With a two-dimensional pattern before him, Martin proceeded
methodically and quickly to reconstruct this with blocks. But in assembling
pictures of objects from parts, with no model before him, he had appreciable
difficulty and sometimes failed to see that some part was upside down. There
was however no lack of determination or perseverance in trying to complete
the tasks nor any sign of frustration or anger when he failed to do so.

He was verbally most fluent and made good use of his excellent vocabulary.
Syntax was perfectly in keeping with his age and background. But articulation
revealed some defects. He mispronounced some words, transposing consonants
occasionally and sometimes used "f" for "th." His parents and his infant
school teacher had noted articulatory defects earlier but these were now slight.
He could not, after many trials, say "preliminary" although he knew the word.
His infant school teacher had also commented on some difficulty in distinguishing certain sounds. On examination, the number of errors Martin made on a
test of auditory discrimination was within normal limits, but even after repetition he failed to distinguish "th" from "f" and "th" from "v."

On a test of visual retention, Martin's performance was well outside the
normal range for his age and IQ. His errors were largely those of rotation and
inaccurate reproduction. He was right-handed, right-eyed and right-footed.
This was a highly intelligent boy with marked inequalities of level in different
areas of function.

Although said to read well, Martin was in fact markedly backward. In reading a prose passage, he used all his considerable linguistic skill and although he misread many words, his comprehension was very good. On a word-reading test without contextual clues, he fared considerably worse. Reading even phonically regular words he would omit letters or syllables or transpose letters or syllables. His spelling age was not quite two years below his chronological age, by no means a great degree of retardation. The true extent of his difficulty becomes apparent only when IQ and oral linguistic skill are considered. His spelling was almost entirely phonetic. He made only one "b" — "d" reversal in the test but mother reported that Martin still frequently reversed "b" and "d" at school.

His parents wrote one year later. His teachers were now much more understanding about the boy's very genuine difficulties. Martin had made some progress but a recent report from school indicated that while general knowledge was excellent Martin still found difficulty in expressing his thoughts on paper and that the bad spelling was a great handicap.

Is this a minor problem? "Minor" is a relative term. Compared with those who can barely read, Martin might almost be said to have no problem. But to Martin and his parents, this is little comfort. Martin is a highly intelligent lad, clearly of University calibre and he himself would like to go to University one day. His reading is likely to continue to improve and it is improbable, even if inaccuracies in reading persist, that these will hold him back appreciably. But the writing difficulty may well persist. It would be wrong because of this to deny to Martin and the many like him the opportunity to develop their other considerable talents.

Margaret, Simon and Donald: a Family

A few families in which more than one child was dyslexic were examined at the Centre. Unaffected as well as affected siblings were examined to discover whether the dyslexics showed any specific features which might distinguish them from the others. Such a family of two boys and a girl is described below. The younger boy and the girl were dyslexic. Three cousins were also severely dyslexic. The elder boy of the family examined had had no difficulty in learning to read, write or spell, but his performance in both reading and spelling spelling revealed uncertainties which were of interest in view of the family background.

Both parents were highly educated. Neither had had any difficulty in learning to read or write but Father was a very slow reader and was left-handed.

Margaret

Margaret was 11½ years of age. Although of bright normal intelligence, she was reading and spelling at a level four years below her chronological age. She had been sent to a small private school of high academic standard just before her fifth birthday. Margaret did not learn to read there, was ridiculed and became aggressive and difficult. She was removed to a junior school. She was referred with full parental agreement and support to the Child Guidance Clinic, where she received much help. She became very much less disturbed but despite some help with reading made very slow progress.

Margaret was a full-term baby, born with the umbilical cord round her neck. There were no complications following the birth. She was a little late

in walking and slow in learning to talk. Articulation was poor and she had
had a slight stutter until shortly before going to school. She was slow to grasp
the grammatical structure of language.

When examined, her use of language was still immature. She showed some
tendency to "twist" sounds, for example "thirsty" was pronounced as
"thristy." On the intelligence test her verbal reasoning ability was well above
average but she found the repetition of a sequence of digits difficult. Arithmetic was very poor and the report from school made reference to her considerable difficulty with the subject.

The examination revealed no further deficit, Margaret performing well
within normal limits in all areas of function explored. She was right-handed,
right-eyed and right-footed.

Despite improvement in her general behaviour, it was clear from both our
examination and the report from school that Margaret was much frustrated
by her inability to read and write. At school it was recognized that she was a
bright child and that she was much handicapped by the dyslexia. But although
Margaret's need for considerable help was acknowledged, there were staff
shortages and her teacher was now at a loss to know how to help.

Simon

Simon was nearly 10 years old but had barely begun to read and write. He too
was of bright normal intelligence. Unlike Margaret, he was sent to an Infant/
Junior school at 5 years of age. On transfer from the Infant to the Junior
Department, it was evident that Simon's complete inability to read required
investigation so he was examined by the local educational psychologist. Subsequen
Simon was given much help both within the school and at the Child Guidance
Clinic, but with little success. He had always been a quiet, rather timid child
and Mother noted that as he grew older and became very aware of his learning
difficulty he had become more withdrawn. At the time of the examination he
presented as a very quiet, inhibited little boy who, though co-operative,
showed none of the enthusiasm shown by most children when given the
"puzzles" and "games" which constitute much of our examination.

Simon's birth history was unremarkable. He was late in walking and very
slow in learning to talk. He had had difficulty in pronouncing some sounds
and slight defects were still present on examination. His use of language had
been and still was poor for age and background. Mother noted that he had
always been a rather clumsy child. On examination, motor co-ordination was
well below the standard appropriate to his age. Like Margaret he was right-
handed, right-eyed and right-footed.

Simon exhibited a slight difficulty in discriminating speech sounds but no
hearing loss. There were remarkable similarities between Margaret and Simon
on the intelligence test. Both children achieved their highest scores on the
tests of verbal reasoning with Vocabulary at a lower level. Their lowest scores
related to Arithmetic and Digit Span. The discrepancy between Simon's
highest and lowest subtest scores was greater than his sister's. Simon was
receiving as much help as the school and clinic could give but he was, none
the less, a depressed child making little if any headway in reading.

Donald

Donald aged 13 years presented an entirely different picture. He was a very
bright boy in a top stream at school. At no time had there been concern over

his reading, writing or spelling. His success was a complicating factor in this family for clearly he overshadowed his younger brother and sister, their difficulties being accentuated by comparison.

Donald's early history was uneventful. He walked and spoke early. Like his brother and sister, he had stuttered slightly when he began to speak but only for a short period. No language difficulties had been noted and none were observed during the examination.

Donald gave no evidence of difficulty on any of the tests administered. The physical examination was negative. The report from school indicated that English was Donald's weakest subject and that his spelling was rather unreliable. His reading age was found to be 15 months in advance of his chronological age but he unexpectedly stumbled over some words. Spelling was slightly below the reading level. Donald's performance during the spelling test was interesting. The easier words he wrote correctly and fluently. Towards the end of the word list he showed great hesitation. He would scribble a word in the margin, realize it was incorrectly spelled, score it out and try again. This was repeated several times. Ultimately some words were correct, others wrong. Sometimes he gave up. Although reading and spelling were in advance of chronological age, an even better performance might have been expected in view of his very high intelligence, his use of language and his background.

There was no history of behavioural disturbance. Indeed, in his report, Donald's headmaster commented more than once that he was a "very normal boy."

Although very different in temperament, Margaret and Simon show certain similarities. Delays in walking and talking and an early slight stutter were common to both. Their use of grammar was not commensurate with age and background. Simon's deficits were more extensive, involving also motor incoordination. Apart from an early slight stutter, Donald showed none of the features shared by his brother and sister. The two dyslexic children alone had developed behaviour problems. One child had become difficult and aggressive, the other withdrawn. These behavioural problems had received most attention. While help had also been given with reading, the reading difficulty was regarded as secondary to the emotional disturbance and treated accordingly. But both children remained severely dyslexic even after treatment.

The problems and difficulties presented by these children are many and various. The children differ with regard to background, intelligence and degree of retardation. Most have received considerable help, but as their difficulties were misdiagnosed the help has not been of the right kind.

All except Donald experienced considerable difficulty in learning to read and/or to spell, a difficulty that was striking by contrast with other learning abilities. Common to all are findings, on full examination, of delays and deficits other than those of reading and spelling. Some of these are likely to contribute to the reading difficulty, others may not. But in the light of background and history, they show developmental anomalies which support the concept of a constitutional disorder.

2

Historical Review

Among those who accept that terms such as dyslexia and word-blindness are meaningful and relate to a distinct minority of backward readers, there is broad agreement that the disorder is specific and constitutionally determined. Beyond such general agreement, however, opinion is still divided as to precise symptomatology and aetiology. Many features suggestive of developmental anomalies have been found to occur in association with a specific reading disability but no single pattern of disabilities has yet been identified. Several explanatory hypotheses relating to aetiology have been advanced, some postulating genetic factors, others neurological damage. Each hypothesis is supported by the results of investigations previously carried out but opinion is still sharply divided as to whether or not a term such as specific dyslexia should be applied only to reading disorders of genetic origin.

It would be impossible within the confines of this volume to refer to all the investigations made during the last seventy years. However, an attempt is made to include studies which illustrate the main schools of thought and which provide the theoretical background to our present investigation.

Terminology

Since congenital word-blindness was first described, many alternative terms have been coined, such as congenital symbolamblyopia, congenital typholexia, congenital alexia, amnesia visualis verbalis, analfabetia partialis and bradylexia (Rabinovitch *et al.*, 1954). Not surprisingly, such terms were discarded almost as soon as they had been invented. Occasionally encountered is Orton's (1937) "strephosymbolia," which literally means "twisting of symbols." Today more commonly used are specific dyslexia, developmental dyslexia, specific developmental dyslexia, congenital dyslexia, word-blindness and congenital word-blindness. The Orton Society in the United States previously used the term "Specific Language Disability." Although these terms are sometimes used interchangeably, as their very multiplicity might suggest, there is a multiplicity of notions about the characteristics and aetiology of the disorders they describe.

The word "dyslexia" is literally translated "defective language" but is generally interpreted as "defective reading." It could therefore be applied to

8

all backward readers and is sometimes loosely so applied, but such usage vitiates its value in distinguishing some backward readers from others.

The term "specific dyslexia" is sometimes restricted to describing familial or genetically determined reading disorders (Critchley, 1964; Crosby, 1968). In this study, the use of this term is not so restricted and for simplicity it is used interchangeably with "dyslexia."

Early History

It has long been recognized that the ability to read, and to learn to read, may be impaired by frank brain damage manifested by clear-cut neurological deficits. Indeed it was the discovery that the reading process could be impaired by brain damage or disease which led to the investigation of neurological anomalies in children with severe difficulties in learning to read. Critchley (1964) presents a fascinating account of this early discovery. Briefly, it was noted with increasing frequency from the 1860s onwards, that some patients who had suffered brain injury or cerebral vascular accident lost the ability to read, usually, though not invariably, in conjunction with loss of speech (aphasia). In 1877 a German physician, Kussmaul, noted that the ability to read might be lost although sight, intellect and speech were unaffected. He invented the term "word-blind." As further similar cases were reported it was observed that there appeared to be two types of word-blindness. In one, the patients could not read but they could write; in the other they could neither read nor write. Post-mortem examinations of the brains of some of these patients revealed lesions, softenings or haemorrhages in the occipito-parietal region of the left cerebral hemisphere.

In 1895 a paper by an eye specialist in Glasgow, James Hinshelwood, was published in *The Lancet* on "Word-Blindness and Visual Memory." This prompted Dr Pringle Morgan (1896) a general practitioner and school doctor, to report the case of Percy aged 14 years. Percy was bright, healthy and of a good family. He was quite good at arithmetic but had an apparently isolated difficulty in learning to read and to write which was seriously interfering with his education. Orally he could more than hold his own in class but when asked to write "Carefully winding the string round the peg," Percy wrote "Calfully winder the strung rond the pag." In the absence of any history of injury or illness, Morgan concluded that this must be a case of congenital word-blindness.

A little later, a School Medical Officer in Bradford, Dr James Kerr (1897), drew attention to several healthy intelligent children who presented a picture similar to Percy. Hinshelwood continued to collect data on cases of what had now come to be called "congenital word-blindness." His monographs *Letter-Word- and Mind-Blindness* and *Congenital Word-Blindness* were published in 1900 and 1917 respectively. Hinshelwood, as did Morgan, attributed the condition to the maldevelopment of the left angular gyrus. Further cases were described by Nettleship (1901), Thomas (1905), Fisher (1905, 1910), Stephenson (1907), Rutherfurd (1909). Stephenson's report of six cases affecting three generations of one family was a forerunner of later studies suggesting that a genetic factor is involved. Fisher (1910) thought that "word-blindness" could be due to cerebral damage and suggested that birth injury might be a predisposing factor.

Following Burt's investigations into backwardness with their emphasis on environmental and psychogenic factors, interest in congenital word-blindness waned. In the United States, Samuel T. Orton, a psychiatrist and neurologist, observed several characteristic phenomena occurring in intelligent neurologically normal children with a specific reading and writing disorder (Orton, 1925, 1928, 1937). These included left-handedness and more particularly mixed-handedness or ambilaterality which Orton called "Motor Intergrading"; frequent reversals in both reading and writing; abnormal clumsiness; some difficulty in understanding spoken language in the absence of deafness; and some difficulty in using language. The tendency to reverse letters and transpose the order of letters was so marked that he invented the term "strephosymbolia" to describe the difficulty.

In Orton's day there was thought to be a direct crossed relationship between the dominant hand and the cerebral hemisphere subserving speech and language, that is, the dominant hemisphere. In right-handed individuals, the left cerebral hemisphere is dominant and in the left-handed, the right hemisphere. In those of indeterminate hand preference, neither hemisphere is dominant. Orton thought that the learning difficulties in oral and written language occurring in otherwise normal children might be explained by a genetically-determined failure of one hemisphere to assume a dominant role in mediating speech and language function. The reversal of letters and confusion over the order of letters and sounds could also be explained by a failure of one hemisphere to become dominant. He assumed that memory images are stored in both hemispheres, in the perceived direction in the dominant and in the opposite or mirrorwise direction in the non-dominant hemisphere. When cerebral dominance is not established, difficulty would be experienced in selecting the correctly orientated memory image or sequence of memory images resulting in the reversals and transpositions he had observed to be so common.

The relationship between the dominant hand and the cerebral hemisphere subserving speech and language is, however, far from clear. It is the left cerebral hemisphere which appears to be dominant in most people, including the left-handed (Humphrey and Zangwill, 1952; Penfield and Roberts, 1959; Espir and Russell, 1961). Exceptions are found and it would appear that the cerebral organization of language is less predictable among those of left- or mixed-handedness, in whom right or bilateral speech representation is more common than in the right-handed (Zangwill, 1960, Milner *et al.,* 1964). In some cases left- or mixed-handedness and right or bilateral speech representation are associated with early brain injury (Penfield and Roberts, 1959).

Current Concepts

At a meeting of the World Federation of Neurologists' Research Group on Dyslexia and World Illiteracy, held in Dallas, Texas, in April 1968, Specific Developmental Dyslexia was defined as: "A disorder manifested by difficulty in learning to read despite conventional instruction, adequate intelligence, and socio-cultural opportunity. It is dependent upon fundamental cognitive disabilities which are frequently of constitutional origin."

The distinction between specific developmental dyslexia and other forms of reading backwardness is made clear by Rabinovitch (1968). He classified reading disability as falling into three types depending on aetiology, and the majority of those using the term specific dyslexia would agree that it corresponds to the first. The types are: (1) A primary retardation in which learning to read is impaired without definite evidence of brain damage from the history or as revealed by neurological examination. The defect lies in the capacity to deal with letters and words as symbols, appearing to reflect a basically disturbed pattern of neural organization. (2) Reading retardation secondary to brain injury in which the capacity to learn to read is impaired by frank brain damage as manifested by clear-cut neurologic deficits. The picture is similar to dyslexia in adults resulting from brain injury and is thought to be due to prenatal toxicity, birth trauma or anoxia, encephalitis or head injury. (3) Reading retardation secondary to environmental factors in which the capacity to learn to read is intact but is given insufficient opportunity for the child to achieve a reading level appropriate to his mental age.

As Rabinovitch points out, children do not always fall neatly into one or other of these groups. While exogenous factors may be clearly present, an extended examination may reveal specific impairments suggestive of a primary retardation. Again the distinction between unequivocal neurological deficits and minor degrees of neurological dysfunction hinges only too often upon the observer's interpretation.

Ingram (1964) distinguishes two types of dyslexia, one found in individuals with evidence of brain injury on history or examination, the other in those without a history or clinical findings suggestive of brain injury. Among the latter are some without a family history of speech defects, or reading or writing difficulty and others with a family history of speech defect, or reading or writing difficulty and often of ambidexterity, sinistrality and twinning. It is doubtful whether any would describe the reading difficulties associated with cerebral palsy or hemiplegia, for example, as a specific dyslexia. But as Ingram points out, there are many cases where the evidence of brain damage is less obvious, cases which exhibit syndromes of "minimal brain dysfunction." The consensus of medical opinion (Bax and Mac Keith, 1963) is against inferring brain injury from such syndromes but this again is frequently a matter of fine clinical judgement.

Critchley (1964) regards any theory of minimal brain damage as unconvincing as it fails to take account of the factor of inheritance and also disregards the frequent absence of neurological deficit even after the most rigorous search. He points out that "the plasticity of the nervous system in the young might be expected to compensate for the effects of any circumscribed lesion of very early appearance."

Genetic transmission

In Scandinavia, a narrower concept of specific dyslexia has been evolved. Word-blindness has been recognized for many years and the Ordblind Institutet in Copenhagen was founded in 1936 by Edith Norrie, herself word-blind, as a teaching centre for word-blind children. Concepts of congenital word-blindness had assumed from the first some form of hereditary transmission. Hallgren's study (1950) of the case and family histories of 276 children with a history of early and prolonged reading difficulty resulted in more direct evidence of an hereditary factor. In 88 per cent there was evidence of a reading disability in the immediate family of each child. Hallgren identified a primary reading disability and suggested that this was inherited as a unitary Mendelian dominant trait. However, since a reading disability may arise from so many causes, it cannot be assumed that a reported familial difficulty is necessarily evidence of genetic origin.

More convincing evidence comes from the study of uniovular and binovular twins. Hermann (1959) assembled three such studies, one of Hallgren's and two of Norrie's. Altogether there were 12 pairs of uniovular twins and in all there was complete concordance regarding dyslexia. Of the 33 pairs of binovular twins concordance was found in only 11 pairs. The emphasis on genetic transmission is reflected in Hermann's definition of specific dyslexia as "a defective capacity for acquiring, at the normal time, a proficiency in reading and writing corresponding to average performance; the deficiency is dependent upon constitutional factors (heredity), is often accompanied by difficulties with other symbols (numbers, musical notation, etc.), it exists in absence of intellectual defect or of defects of the sense organs which might retard the normal accomplishment of those skills, and in the absence of past or present appreciable inhibitory influences in the internal and external environments."

Maturational Lag

The examination of dyslexic children commonly reveals many associated difficulties. Many investigators have been impressed by the multiplicity of these in young dyslexic children and the infrequency with which they occur in older children. Critchley (1964) notes that many dyslexic children, particularly those who are highly intelligent, show spontaneous improvement, in reading and writing skills, even without much help, usually at about the age of puberty.

De Hirsch, with many years of experience at a Paediatric Language Disorder Clinic, was struck by the relatively immature level in perceptuomotor and language skill shown by children of adequate or good intelligence who later experienced severe difficulties in learning to read and write. She, with her colleagues (de Hirsch, Jansky and Langford, 1966) administered a battery of 37 tests to 53 kindergarten children. Performance was related to levels of reading and spelling two and one half years later. Twenty-seven of the tests involved tasks on which improvement with age was noted and 76 per cent of these correlated significantly with subsequent reading scores as against 17 per cent of those which were not sensitive to maturation. Twelfth among the predictive measures was IQ and the correlation between IQ and spelling was low. An apparent maturational lag may of course be due to lack of opportunity and experience, but, as will be seen below, many "lags" are remarkably persistent and suggestive of inherent defect.

The results of many experiments by Birch and his colleagues (Birch, 1962) have demonstrated certain sequences in the maturation of perceptual abilities through which young children explore and learn about their world and which are most relevant to learning to read. The child receives information through all his senses but at different stages of development different senses predominate, at first the sensory systems of touch and movement, followed by vision and hearing. Attention can be paid only to a limited number of the sensations constantly being received and the sensory system which predominates will partly determine to which aspects of his environment a child will respond and which aspects remain in the background.

Information received through one sensory system is not automatically transmitted to or integrated with information received through another system. A child has to learn to associate the tick of a clock with the sight of a clock so that when he hears the tick he will associate this with the object he has seen. Ultimately the idea of "clock" will be triggered by either the sound or sight of a clock. The ability to integrate information from different sensory systems becomes evident as the child matures and develops normally. But children show wide variations in the rate at which development takes place and some children when they enter school may not have reached the stage where intersensory integrations are easily formed, for example, between the words they hear and use and the visual symbols by which words and sounds are represented. Birch and Belmont (1964) have shown that many retarded readers have difficulty in tasks which require the child to select from a number of visual patterns that one which matches a pattern of sounds.

Particularly relevant to learning to read is the ability to analyse words into their component sounds and to synthesize or blend sounds and syllables into whole words. Maturational factors in the acquisition of these skills have been demonstrated by two studies. Leroy-Bussion and Dupessey (1969) examined the ability to blend sounds of young children of average intelligence, aged from 4 years to 6 years 11 months and found that this ability increased with age and that the rate of increase was correlated with IQ. By 6 years of age, most children could blend sounds, but some revealed a specific difficulty in carrying out this task. These findings complement Bruce's (1964) study of the capacity of children aged 5 years 1 month to 7 years 6 months, to make a simple phonetic analysis of the spoken word, for example, to say what word would be left if "c" were removed from "clock." Children were unable to do this until a mental age of 7 years had been reached. The type of instruction given at school and the length of time the children had been at school were also important factors. Bright children, who had been at school for a short time only, failed on the tasks. So also did those who had received much phonic instruction, until they had reached a mental age of 7

Reading, writing and spelling are very complex acts and require competence in the understanding and use of language, in the ability to distinguish one sound from another, one shape from another, be this a single letter or a complex word pattern. The child has to learn to recognize these patterns and to recall them, accurately reproducing the letters of a word in correct sequence. Associations between sounds and shapes must be formed. Fine control of hand and eye and co-ordination between hand and eye are needed. These skills are still maturing when children go to school. Children differ widely in the rate at which they develop and sometimes, in the individual child, there are marked variations in the rate at which different skills mature. Discrepant levels of function within the individual child may be due to environmental conditions which do not provide the opportunity to develop particular skills or they may possibly be related to an unusually delayed maturation of a part of the brain (Rutter, Tizard and Whitmore, 1970). Marked delays in the acquisition of isolated functions may also be found in brain-injured children and when they are found in dyslexic children in conjunction with signs of neurological dysfunction, the question of brain damage is raised.

Neurological Dysfunction

The reading disability which may be found in children with manifest signs of neurological abnormality is not a specific dyslexia. However, in many cases of specific reading disability, minor or "soft" neurological signs have been elicited. Evidence of neurological dysfunction has emerged from a number of studies of dyslexic children.

Cohn (1961) reported, in a study of 46 dyslexic children aged 7 to 10 years and 130 children with no reading difficulty, significant differences in right/left orientation, the evaluation of double simultaneous tactile stimuli, knee-jerk reflexes, the Babinski sign, motor co-ordination, the mechanics of speech and EEG patterns. Signs of neurological dysfunction were still present after two years when 29 of the dyslexic children were re-examined. This picture of persisting neurological signs, albeit using different indices, is echoed by two studies by Silver and Hagin (1960, 1964). A battery of tests, psychological and neurological, was administered on two occasions with an interval of ten to twelve years to 24 dyslexics, 3 girls and 21 boys. In their first study, Silver and Hagin identified three groups of specific reading disability: (1) a developmental group; (2) an "organic" group with evidence of structural organic defect; (3) a very small group showing no perceptual deficits or signs. In the follow-up study, 15 of this sample were deemed to be adequate readers and they tended to come from the "developmental" group and to be less severely retarded as children. The "organic" group showed less improvement than the others and their specific perceptual deficits and lack of clear cerebral dominance tended to persist.

Neurological abnormalities were identified by Kinsbourne and Warrington (1963 *b*) in a group of 13 dyslexics referred for a neurological opinion on account of an apparently selective reading impairment. The children were selected on the basis of a difference of 20 points or more between the Verbal and Performance sections of the Wechsler Intelligence Scale for Children (WISC). Among those with the lower Performance IQ, there was a higher incidence of neurological abnormality and also of right/left disorientation and finger agnosia. Histories suggestive of birth injury were more common in this group.

Boshes and Myklebust (1964) included a neurological examination in their investigation of the learning disorders of 85 children from 7 to 18 years with an IQ of at least 90, no hearing or visual defects, no obvious cerebral palsy or emotional disturbance. Suspect or positive neurological signs were found in 44 children. Unlike the previously quoted study, Boshes and Myklebust found that the significant associations with neurological dysfunction occurred mainly with auditory-verbal rather than with visual or nonverbal behaviour. They also noted lower intertest correlations with chronological age among those with positive neurological signs, suggesting that the growth expecte with increasing age is less evident where neurological deficits are found.

It is difficult to determine to what extent neurological dysfunction represents actual damage to the nervous system in the absence of gross neurological deficits and evidence of predisposing conditions is desirable. Perinatal conditions have been implicated in the studies of Kawi and Pasamanick (1958) Prechtl (1962), Kinsbourne and Warrington (1963 *b*), Lucas, Rodin and Simson (1965) and Lyle (1970) and these in conjunction with motor, neurological and learning deficits strongly suggest neurological damage. Zangwill (1962 *b*) pointed out that the prognosis is likely to be different depending upon the aetiology of the dysfunction and this is supported by the studies of Silver and Hagin (1964) and of Cohn (1961).

Cerebral Dominance

The atypical patterns of neurological organization and development postulated by Orton have been referred to. As indicated earlier the association between the dominant side of the body and cerebral dominance is not so direct as was once thought, but the studies quoted by Zangwill (1960) on hand preference in relation to localized cortical lesions make it reasonable to suppose that the development of differential cerebral hemispheric function and individual patterns of handedness are in some way associated. Evidence relating to the incidence of left-handedness or more particularly indeterminate handedness in retarded readers is conflicting. Many studies have revealed no differences in the proportion of atypical patterns of laterality between unselected retarded readers and control groups (Gates and Bond, 1936; Witty and Kopel, 1936; Smith, 1950; Hilman, 1956; Belmont and Birch, 1965). On the other hand, where high frequencies have been reported, the subjects were mostly children referred to hospitals for neurological investigation and in this sense "selected" (Ettlinger and Jackson, 1955; Ingram and Reid, 1956; Galifret-Granjon, 1959; Zangwill, 1960). Affected children have been more commonly ill-lateralized than strongly left-handed as Shearer (1968) also found. The present writer (Naidoo, 1961), in a study of 5-year-old children selected solely on the basis of hand preference, found that 20 ill-lateralized children, matched for age, sex and school with 20 strongly left-handed and 20 strongly right-handed children, were significantly inferior with regard to verbal intelligence. Histories of slow speech development were more frequent among the ill-lateralized children. Zangwill (1960) was impressed by the frequency with which retarded speech development, defects of spatial perception, clumsiness and related indications of defective maturation occurred in ill-lateralized dyslexic children. In discussing why only some ill-lateralized children should have reading difficulties, Zangwill (1962 b) put forward three possible explanations: (1) that poorly developed laterality and the reading retardation, when occurring together, may be the effects of an actual cerebral lesion; (2) that, in the absence of neurological lateralizing signs, a genetic factor controlling handedness and cerebral dominance may be involved and associated with slow maturation: (3) that those lacking strong and consistent lateral preferences are particularly vulnerable to stress such as that of a minimal birth injury.

Summary

Although the current concepts of dyslexia have been outlined under the specific headings of genetic factors, maturational lag, neurological dysfunction and cerebral dominance, these need not be mutually exclusive. Genetic factors may underlie the maturational lag, neurological dysfunction and patterns of atypical cerebral dominance. It is clear, too, that evidence of genetic factors in the form of positive familial histories is lacking in many cases of specific dyslexia. Opinion is still divided as to the extent to which pathological neurological dysfunction should be included among the aetiological factors of dyslexia. Myklebust and Johnson (1962), defining dyslexia as "an inability to read normally as a result of a dysfunction in the brain," recognize that this may occur as the result of disease, accident or on the basis of heredity. Many British investigators, including Critchley (1964) and Gooddy (1967), would emphatically exclude children with evidence of clear neurological impairment

But even when grosser neurological signs are excluded there is evidence from a number of studies of signs which point to a minor grade of neurological impairment. While the interpretation of these in terms of minimal brain damage is still controversial (Bax and Mac Keith, 1963) the possibility that they may be of pathological significance cannot be ignored.

Some definitions of dyslexia stress the presence of "adequate" intelligence and this is usually interpreted as meaning of at least average intelligence. It is obvious that if aetiological factors such as genetic transmission and neurological dysfunction are implicated, specific dyslexia can occur at all levels of intelligence. The crucial identifying feature is then the presence of a specific learning difficulty, the major presenting symptom being a difficulty in learning to read relative to the learning of other skills. Again, as Rabinovitch *et al.* (1954) Vernon (1962) and others have pointed out, specific dyslexia may be aggravated by adverse environmental factors and/or emotional maladjustment and just because these are present one should not conclude that there is no constitutional basis for the dyslexia.

Other Learning Disorders Associated with Dyslexia

While there is much evidence to support the concept of specific dyslexia as a constitutionally determined disorder, critics of its existence frequently point to a failure so far to identify a single condition of single aetiology within a characteristic syndrome of signs and symptoms. Not only does there appear to be more than one cause of the disorder but previous studies have identified many other minor difficulties occurring in association with dyslexia, which vary from child to child and which seem to present no clear picture of what dyslexia is.

A disturbance in the appreciation of right and left has been found to be common in dyslexic children (Harris, 1957; Belmont and Birch, 1965; Rutter, Tizard and Whitmore, 1970). Hermann (1959) postulated that a right/left confusion is one of the primary factors underlying specific dyslexia and gives rise to errors of rotation and reversal.

Piaget (1928) identified three stages in the evolution of concepts of right and left. During the first stage, from 5 to 8 years, right and left can be identified in relation to the child's own body. Between 8 to 11 years, the child learns to project notions of right and left to people and objects facing him. Finally, at about 11 or 12 years of age, concepts of right and left are so completely understood that a child can reliably identify right/left relationships between a number of objects. A right/left confusion, inappropriate to the age of a child, may be a sign of developmental delay. The confusion is thought to reflect a disturbed appreciation of direction but, as Benton (1958) pointed out, it may also reflect a disturbance in the use of language.

Delayed speech development, and disorders of speech and language are reported to be common among dyslexic children. A history of late speech development was found by Ingram and Mason (1965) and by Debray (1968) and defective articulation by Monroe (1932) and Doehring (1968). The Isle of Wight Survey revealed that delay in the onset of speech, articulatory disorders and an immature use of language occurred more frequently among children with a specific reading retardation than among their controls (Rutter, Tizard and Whitmore, 1970).

The ability to discriminate between sounds which are similar, for example "th" and "f," "a" and "e," is poor in some retarded readers (Wepman, 1960; Clark, 1970).

The successful blending of sounds is to some extent dependent upon an ability to retain and to reproduce a sequence of sounds in correct order. Several investigators have shown that the recall of sentences or of a sequence of orally presented digits may be defective (Burt, 1937; Myklebust and Johnson, 1962; Doehring, 1968).

Speech and language development are closely related to environmental conditions. The child in residential care, deprived of a normal family life, the child who is rejected by his parents and the child who grows up in an extremely unstimulating home are likely to be linguistically and educationally retarded (Kellmer Pringle, 1965). However, Mittler's (1969) investigation of the language abilities of 4-year-old twins, identical and fraternal, indicates that the development of language skills is also influenced by hereditary factors. The speech and language disorders found in many children with a specific reading disability may be an effect of or a precursor to the reading difficulty. They may be both cause and effect.

The use of the term "congenital *word-blindness*" was based on the postulate that the condition was due to an inability to perceive, store and recall the visual images of words (Hinshelwood, 1917).

The ability to discriminate letter and word shapes is clearly of major importance in learning to read but the numerous studies quoted by Vernon (1958) indicate that difficulties in visual discrimination *per se* are not common among backward readers. Difficulties in discriminating between shapes differing in orientation are more commonly reported (Fildes, 1921; Galifret-Granjon and Ajuriaguerra, 1951; Tjossem, Hansen and Ripley, 1962; Doehring, 1968; Lyle, 1969). The difficulty has been thought to reflect immaturity or defect in the development of the child's ability to appreciate spatial relations (Krise, 1952). However Hendrickson and Muehl (1962) raise the question of whether, in discriminating between "b" and "d," for example, the problem is one of perceiving a difference or of realizing that differences in orientation are important. Lyle and Goyen (1968) who found visual perceptual deficits but no reversal tendencies in a group of retarded readers of average intelligence, attributed reversal tendencies to faulty verbal labelling, a suggestion which receives some support from Asso and Wyke's (1970) study of 60 young children of 4½ to 7½ years.

Retarded readers are frequently reported to perform poorly on tasks requiring the copying of figures, essentially visuo-motor tasks (Lachmann, 1960; Galifret-Granjon, 1952; Debray, 1968). Brenner and Gillman (1966) have provided normative data on a range of visuo-motor tasks in 810 children, 427 boys and 383 girls, aged 7 years 10 months to 9 years 2 months. On the basis of individual total score deviations from total sample means, 144 children were divided into those with high and those with low scores. Fifty-six children of good intelligence with an apparently specific visuo-motor impairment were identified. In none of these was school achievement commensurate with verbal ability. Although reading reasonably well, difficulties in arithmetic and spelling were common. A further characteristic was clumsiness of gait or of movement or of fine motor control.

The ability to reproduce visual patterns from memory would seem to play an important part in spelling, particularly in the spelling of phonetically irregular words where sound alone is an insufficient cue to the written form. Lyle (1969) recently found that the recall of visual patterns was significantly poorer in retarded readers of at least average intelligence. He found, moreover, that the retarded readers produced distortions similar to those made by brain-injured patients but not to the same extent. Lyle suggested that such deficits reflect a minimal cerebral dysfunction and in a later publication (1970) reported a relationship between birth variables and visual perceptual and perceptual-motor skills.

Reading and spelling not only require competence in speech, language, visual and motor skills but rest ultimately on associations made between them. In trying to determine why these complex integrative tasks are so difficult for some children most investigators have been concerned with the examination of the more discrete functions involved. That the defect might be rather in the co-ordination of auditory, visual and tactile sensory patterns is suggested by the work of Birch and Belmont (1964), Beery (1967) and Kahn and Birch (1968).

Is Specific Dyslexia a Single Condition?

So far it has not been possible to isolate common distinguishing features which would incontrovertibly identify specific dyslexia as a single condition. It is clear that all children described as dyslexic, whatever the criteria, do not present the same signs and symptoms. It has therefore been suggested that there may be different varieties of dyslexia recognizable by different patterns of disability. If this is so then, as Kinsbourne and Warrington (1963 b) point out, test results may fail to reach significance because samples are likely to include more than one type of disability.

Ingram (1964) suggests that three sub-categories can be identified on the basis of the nature of the difficulties presented:

   (1) those with visuo-spatial difficulties;
   (2) those with speech sound difficulties;
   (3) those with correlating difficulties.

When reading, the first group may fail to recognize letters or groups of letters, tend to guess words from shape rather than context, confuse reversible letters, transpose letters in syllables, syllables in words and words in phrases. They may read backwards. When writing, there is a difficulty in reproducing letters and groups of letters correctly. Letters are reversed and shapes confused. Transpositions of letter, syllable and word order are common.

The second group is characterized by difficulties in synthesizing words from component sounds, in understanding words and sentences correctly read. When writing, difficulty may occur in breaking words into syllables, in finding words and in constructing sentences.

The third group have difficulty in finding the appropriate speech sounds for individual letters or groups of letters and are unable to recall the visual form of sounds in writing. Ingram comments that such difficulties appear to be more marked with monosyllabic words.

More recently, Johnson and Myklebust (1967) have described two forms of specific dyslexia based on differing symptomatology, visual dyslexia and

auditory dyslexia. The visual dyslexic's difficulties are typified by disturbances in learning via the visual modality. Commonly found are difficulties
in visual discrimination particularly of complex patterns, letter reversals and
inversions, disorders in perceiving and reproducing visual sequences. Visual
retention is poor and the rate of perception slow. Whole word recognition in
reading is faulty and hesitant. Some children in this group are rather clumsy
and poor at games. The auditory dyslexic, on the other hand, finds difficulty
in analysing words into constituent sounds or syllables and in synthesizing
sounds and syllables into meaningful whole words. He has difficulty in perceiving common sound units and thus may fail to identify words which rhyme
or to produce these on request. There may be some difficulty in auditory
discrimination particularly when short vowels and consonant blends are
involved. The reproduction of sounds and words may be defective and silent
reading easier than reading aloud. The ability to reproduce a sequence of
sounds may be poor both with regard to the span of the sequence and its
order. The writing of these children is neat and they may be good at games
and handicrafts.

There are many similarities between Johnson and Myklebust's visual
dyslexics and Ingram's group exhibiting visuo-spatial difficulties and also
between the auditory dyslexic and those with speech-sound difficulties.
However it would be misleading to suggest that dyslexics fall neatly into one
or other of the categories described above. Groups, such as those described
above, reflect discrepant modality patterning, patterns of strengths and
weaknesses occurring in different areas of function. De Hirsch *et al.* (1966)
found that only 10 of 53 subjects aged 5 years 8 months to 6 years 1 month,
exhibited such discrepancies. Seven of these exhibited deficits in the visual-
perceptual and visuo-motor areas, the remaining 3 failed in the auditory-
perceptual and excelled in the visual-perceptual tests. Both the modality
equivalence and the discrepant patterning in De Hirsch's study could well be
related to the age of the subjects. At a later age, at a later stage of maturation
and with further exposure to varied learning situations, the patterns might
have been different.

These recent attempts to identify differing patterns of disability among
dyslexic children are of more than theoretical significance. They are of crucial
importance to the planning of remedial education. A comment made
commonly and necessarily in retrospect is that dyslexic children are
apparently resistant to conventional methods of instruction. This has been
held by some to be due to bad teaching or to emotional resistance (Ilg and
Ames, 1950; Collins, 1961; Daniels, 1962; Burt, 1966). It is just as likely that
the reason for the failure of the children to respond to teaching lies in failure
to elicit and understand the peculiar and specific nature of these children's
difficulties. If there are indeed different sub-groups each presenting different symptoms, then it is unlikely that one method of teaching will be equally
successful with all dyslexics.

The argument that each child's difficulty could be dealt with efficiently
enough by giving due consideration to symptoms alone, is questionable.
Speech and language, for example, may be poorly developed as a result of
environmental linguistic deprivation, genetic endowment, frank brain damage,
emotional disturbance or varying combinations of these. Is one teaching
technique likely to be equally effective in improving speech and language

skills including the written forms, irrespective of the reason for the deficit?
Is the rate of learning likely to be unaffected by the reason for the deficit?
And, other factors being equal, will the levels ultimately achieved be the
same? These are some issues of importance in planning remedial education
and they demand a consideration not only of symptoms but also of
aetiology.

ICAA Conference on Word-Blindness or Specific Developmental Dyslexia — 1962

The controversies surrounding the existence, nature, and causes of specific
dyslexia were clearly demonstrated at the Conference called by the Invalid
Children's Aid Association on Word-Blindness or Specific Developmental
Dyslexia in April 1962 (Franklin, 1962).

The papers presented reflected in the variety of their content some of
the heterogeneity of symptoms and aetiology already described.

Gallagher emphasized the bizarre quality of the reading and writing of
word-blind children, differentiating the brain-injured, the emotionally disturbed and the word-blind. Riis-Vestergaard referred to the speech and
language disorders which may accompany dyslexia, as did Worster-Draught.
Riis-Verstergaard commented upon the difficulty of overcoming congenital
word-blindness completely. De Séchelles indicated something of the variety
of associated disorders which may be found, including communication
disorders, disorders in concepts of time and space, laterality patterns, and the
disorganization of body image. Meredith stressed the fact that all that is
involved in word-blindness is not understood and echoed Vernon's (1962)
plea for more accurate and systematic investigation particularly of individual
cases rather than by large-scale surveys including all types of reading
disability. Critchley drew attention to the presence of the motor, sensory,
visuo-spatial, temporal and linguistic disorders which may accompany a
specific developmental dyslexia. Shankweiler raised some fundamental
questions relating to oral/auditory disturbances, disturbance of form perception, directional sense, immediate memory span and word recognition
and suggested a strategy of dissociation as well as association of symptoms
which might lead to a classification of different forms of dyslexia. Reinhold
indicated the need to distinguish children with congenital dyslexia from other
forms of reading retardation, stressed the presence of the severe spelling
difficulty which is usually more marked than the reading one and indicated
the frequency with which right-left disorientation occurs. Holt, in contrast
to some others, pointed out that word-blindness might occur in children of
any IQ. Miles laid stress on the fact that it was the visual aspect of printed
words which failed to become meaningful in the two cases reported and for
whom a method of teaching had been devised.

Daniels accepted the use of terms like "alexia," "dyslexia" or "word-
blindness" to describe the loss of reading ability following brain lesions, but
was not prepared to subscribe to analogous conditions in children or to accept
a genetic factor in reading disability. He thought that the problem of reading
difficulty lay in the teaching methods adopted and the wide reliance on the
whole-word approach. Much of Daniels's resistance to accepting the concept of
word-blindness seemed to result from his erroneous belief that little can be
done about it.

In the discussions that followed the papers, opinion was divided as to the existence of word-blindness. Most of the opposition to the concept of specific dyslexia was expressed by educational psychologists and was based on several grounds. (1) Retarded readers, whatever one may call them, represent the lower part of the continuum of levels of reading achievement to be found in any normal population. (This may well be so, but concepts based on continua are merely descriptive, offer nothing by way of explanation as to why some individuals should be found at one end and others found at the opposite end and they raise the whole question of what is "normal" variation and what factors contribute to it.) (2) Factors such as poor teaching, unstimulating backgrounds, lack of motivation, severe emotional disturbance and dullness could explain all cases of reading retardation. (This makes nonsense of explanations in terms of a continuum.) (3) The use of labels such as word-blindness or specific developmental dyslexia has an adverse effect on children, parents and teachers because if it is a neurological condition little can be done to help. (This is a most curious attitude. Psychologists and educationists have already risen magnificently to challenges in many fields of special education where biological and neurological disorders are clearly manifest. Why there should be a reluctance to accept and meet a similar challenge in some reading and writing disorders is difficult to understand.)

The variations of symptoms and aetiology discussed by the speakers did not reflect, as Ravenette (1968) would later have it, "contradictory statements of definition." On the contrary, there were broad areas of agreement. Dyslexia is not part of a global learning disorder. It is not primarily due to environmental factors in home or school. It is not due to a severe emotional disturbance. These were negative grounds of general agreement. On the positive side, all were agreed that the disorder is a constitutional one, sometimes genetically determined, and although some speakers placed more emphasis on the presence of particular associated features than did others all were agreed that there were variations in symptomatology. There is no inherent contradiction here but a reflection of imperfect knowledge. Again, medical science is well acquainted with conditions which can affect human beings in clinically different ways. Franklin (1968) sees the problem partly as a clinical one. Drawing an analogy with fever, he points out that at one time, fever itself was a sufficient diagnosis. As differences in clinical pattern, onset, course and associated symptoms were noted, so fevers were subclassified. So it is with reading disorders. Many contributory factors and types of disorder have been identified but problems of further identification remain.

3

The Word Blind Centre for Dyslexic Children and Outline of the Study

At the Invalid Children's Aid Association Conference many recommendations were made. These included a need for further research and Zangwill's view, which was generally supported, was that investigation should be done by workers active in psychology and teaching and that the research should bear upon remedial teaching methods and their outcome. Appropriate facilities for assessment and teaching were urgently needed, as well as opportunity for the special training of teachers.

In the year after this Conference, the ICAA established a centre in their offices in Palace Gate, London, with Dr A. White Franklin as Honorary Medical Director and Dr A. D. Bannatyne as Psychologist. In 1965, with the help of Mr Gordon Piller of the Institute of Child Health, the Centre moved to larger accommodation in Coram's Fields in Guilford Street, where the Centre's staff of psychologists and teachers could be increased. The setting up of the Centre and the research project were made possible by grants from the Children's Research Fund and the City Parochial Foundation.

The initial aims of the Centre were:

(1) To undertake research into the nature and cause of specific reading disability with a view to finding out whether a specific developmental dyslexia could be identified.

(2) To develop a battery of suitable diagnostic tests.

(3) To examine and experiment with various teaching methods and to determine which are the most effective for children with specific dyslexia.

(4) To study the possibility of the predictive screening of young children.

(5) To promote a wider interest among the public, professional bodies and administrators, in the educational problems of dyslexic children.

Children with reading, writing and spelling disorders were accepted for assessment at the Centre, provided they were of at least average intelligence and had no gross neurological defect. Inquiries for assessment came from parents, doctors in private practice, hospitals and school services, psychologists, head and assistant teachers. At first the initial inquiry came usually from the parents, but latterly more than a half of the children examined had been referred directly by professional workers. Parents' requests for assessment had to be supported by referral from a doctor, from the School Psychological

Services or from the child's Head Teacher. Before carrying out an examination at the Centre, a full inquiry was made from the school and from everyone who had examined the child previously. This made possible the exclusion of children of low intelligence and those with cerebral palsy and other recognized neurological disorders. The Centre's purpose was to concentrate on children with as pure a difficulty in reading, writing and spelling as could be found.

Tuition was offered only to a small number of children, selected from the many who were examined. Not all examined were regarded as specifically dyslexic, and children judged to be in need of psychotherapy were not usually accepted for tuition. Especial consideration was given to those with perceptual deficits which seemed to require specialized individually given tuition, to those who were not improving despite remedial teaching locally and to those for whom there was no appropriate provision locally. Although it was mainly children with severe reading difficulties who were accepted for tuition, exception was made in the case of a few children who could read quite well but whose difficulty in writing and spelling hampered their educational progress. Since the children came to the Centre twice a week while attending their normal schools, travelling distance was another factor in selection. Most of the children examined needed help, and whatever the nature of a child's problem, a summary of findings and appropriate recommendations were sent to schools. Children judged suitable were referred to the local School Psychological Service for treatment. It was, however, extremely difficult and often impossible to find help locally for children who read reasonably well but had marked writing and spelling difficulties.

Outline of the Study

There is much evidence to support the concept that some reading disorders have a constitutional basis but there is still a marked reluctance to accept the possibility that constitutional factors may underlie the reading disorders of children who appear to be physically and neurologically normal. A medical examination of children with a reading difficulty is rarely carried out and it is inferred that a child who appears to be physically and neurologically normal *is* so. Emotional disturbance, low IQ, conditions in the home or in the school are common alternative explanations.

Much of the resistance to recognizing the existence of dyslexia appears to be due to an expectation that so definite a term must describe a definitive single condition and to the failure as yet to identify such a condition. Some of the variability of findings from previous studies is due to differences in the criteria used to select samples and to the heterogeneous nature of some of the groups. Would a carefully selected sample of children give evidence of a single syndrome or, as has already been suggested, of different types or sub-groups each with a characteristic pattern of disabilities? A distinction has been made between a genetic dyslexia and one associated with a possibly acquired neurological dysfunction. Opinion is divided as to whether or not a single term such as "specific dyslexia" should be applied to both. On clinical or psychological grounds, can a genetic and an acquired dyslexia be distinguished?

By investigating in some depth a highly selected group of children, an attempt is made to answer these questions. The children were selected as far as possible to exclude those factors commonly associated with and thought to give rise to a difficulty in learning to read and to conform to an acceptable definition of specific dyslexia. In order to allow significant features relating to characteristics and aetiology to emerge from an analysis of the data, it was essential that the criteria for selection should exclude possible significant features.

When the Centre was first set up, the Word Blind Centre's Committee, instead of attempting a definition, laid down certain criteria for the recognition of word-blind children. These were:

Always present:
(1) Reading and spelling considerably behind intelligence.
(2) Inability to deal with symbols forming letters or words and weak retention of symbols.
(3) Bizarre spelling.
(4) Persistent reversal of letters.

Commonly present:
(1) Crossed laterality.
(2) Bizarre and cramped handwriting.
(3) Difficulties with numbers similar to the difficulties with letters.
(4) Weakness in copying diagrams.
(5) Similar difficulties in other members of the family in the same or earlier generations.
(6) Sometimes a secondary emotional disturbance showing itself in physical symptoms which recur frequently and lead to absence from school, which is then blamed for the reading difficulty.

The use of such criteria for selecting children in our investigation into characteristics and aetiology would have prejudged results. Instead a definition similar to Eisenberg's (1962) was employed. For the purpose of selecting children for this investigation, specific dyslexia is defined as a condition causing difficulty in learning to read and to spell in physically normal intelligent children in spite of continuous schooling and in the absence of severe emotional disturbance. This definition was translated into the objective criteria specified in the next chapter.

The limitation of such a definition lies in the implication that the disorder exists only in the absence of certain factors. If specific dyslexia is a congenital or developmentally determined disorder it must surely be found in children at all levels of intelligence and irrespective of home and school conditions. However, it was clear at the outset of this study that our experimental group would not be large enough to examine the effect of low IQ, emotional instability and many adverse home and school conditions.

One feature included in most definitions is missing, namely the assumption that specific dyslexia is a constitutionally or organically determined disorder, an assumption which would either be supported or refuted by the analysis of the data. The experimental group is highly selected not only with regard to the presence of a very specific reading and spelling difficulty but also socio-economically. The majority of children examined at the Centre have come from middle-class backgrounds. Since this was so, many of the variables relating, for example, to developmental history, neurological integrity, motor co-ordination, some aspects of speech and language and familial disorders, would, if found to be present in the experimental group to a significant degree, support the hypothesis that dyslexia is constitutionally determined.

Only boys are included in this study. The ratio of boys to girls examined at the Centre has consistently been 5:1. The number of girls meeting the selection criteria was not large enough to permit of adequate statistical analysis and girls are, therefore, excluded.

The dyslexic boys are divided into two groups. The first exhibits a severe degree of reading and spelling retardation, and the second a severe spelling retardation and a relatively minor degree of reading difficulty. The division of the sample into two groups was made for several reasons. Dyslexia is thought of as an extreme difficulty in learning to read, write and spell. "Extreme" is usually taken to mean that the *degree* of reading retardation is great. Many children taught at the Centre read tolerably well but their writing and spelling constituted a real educational handicap, and it was inordinately difficult if not impossible to improve their writing and spelling beyond a level much too low to enable them to record their knowledge and thoughts on paper in an acceptable form. Such difficulties must also be regarded as extreme. But while very backward readers are at least recognized, the very poor spellers are not. It was almost impossible to find help for the latter outside the Centre.

Very backward readers and those backward to lesser degree seemed to exhibit many similar features. By investigating both groups separately, it was hoped to discover whether or not their disorders were of an essentially similar nature.

Much thought was given to suitable terms to describe the two groups. To have labelled them simply as Group 1 and Group 2 would have made it difficult for the reader to keep in mind their distinguishing features. To have called them "severely dyslexic" and "mildly dyslexic" would have assumed that both groups exhibited a similar condition and that only a difference in its severity distinguished them. Children who have great difficulty in learning to read are identified by their reading difficulty. Their spelling difficulty is usually even greater but the major handicap as far as their education is concerned is the reading problem. The very backward readers are therefore described as Reading Retardates. In those less backward in reading, it is their poor spelling which is the major concern. Although the spelling is in some cases not so poor as that found among the Reading Retardates, the term Spelling Retardate seemed suitably to describe them.

Each experimental group was matched for age and type of school with a similar number of boys unselected for reading and spelling ability.

The data were obtained from a medical and a psychological examination, from parents and schools. Obstetric reports were obtained for most children born in hospital. The information related to family conditions, school conditions, the adjustment of the children in schools, perinatal conditions, early development, physical and neurological status, familial reading, spelling, speech and laterality factors and performance on a battery of tests designed to elicit many of the associated features described by previous investigators.

Where the variables were of a qualitative nature, the hypotheses were concerned with the frequency with which a response occurred. Most of the psychological tests are quantitatively scored and hypotheses pertaining to these have been concerned with differences in average scores. The majority of the tests used were standardized. The clinician is often interested in the numbers of children who perform below a level which test standardization has indicated as normal for age. Therefore, consideration is also given to the numbers of children whose performance places them inside or outside "normal" limits.

The first part of the analysis is aimed at identifying those single variables which distinguish each dyslexic group from its respective control group. If similar other specific learning disabilities, developmental anomalies and aetiological factors were found in both experimental groups, then this would support the hypothesis of a single disorder with its own continuum ranging from severe to mild. Since, apart from selection on similar basic criteria, the two experimental groups were not matched for age, IQ or type of school, they could not be directly compared. In the case of quantitatively scored variables, similarities and differences between the experimental groups themselves have been explored by comparing the size of the difference between the Reading Retardates and their Control group with the size of the difference between the Spelling Retardates and their Control group. Where the difference between the Reading Retardates and their controls differs significantly from the difference between the Spelling Retardates and their controls, this is interpreted as indicating that the two experimental groups are dissimilar with respect to the variable concerned.

The second part of the analysis attempts to identify sub-groups or different forms of dyslexia. Selected variables were submitted to a Cluster Analysis. The programme used allowed groups to emerge from the data themselves without previously formulating hypotheses. If clusters or groups emerged, they could be compared with groups previously described.

4

Subjects and Criteria for Selection

Dyslexic Boys

Boys with severe reading and/or spelling difficulties were selected from those examined at the Word Blind Centre from January 1967 to March 1969. Altogether 271 boys were examined medically and psychologically during the relevant period. The age range was 6 to 13 years, but the problems of identifying a specific reading and spelling difficulty and of finding a battery of tests suitable for such a wide age range led to the decision to restrict the sample to those from 8 years to 12 years 11 months inclusive.

Two groups were selected, Reading Retardates and Spelling Retardates. All met the following criteria:

(1) Full Scale IQ on the Wechsler Intelligence Scale for Children not less than 90 and in no case was the Verbal IQ less than 85.

(2) Physically and grossly neurologically normal on examination by the Honorary Medical Adviser, Dr A. White Franklin, or Dr Macdonald Critchley.

(3) No major absence from school, especially during the first two years and no more than three changes of school, excluding the normal transfer from infant to junior school, for example.

(4) No evidence of severe emotional disturbance on the psychologist's examination of the child and interview with parents, and from the Bristol Social Adjustment Guide completed by the school. A psychiatric examination was not made.

The reading accuracy age of the Reading Retardates is at least two years below chronological age. (The Neale Analysis of Reading Ability Accuracy Age was used for boys of 9 years to 12 years 11 months and the reading age on Schonell's Graded Word Reading Test for the 8-year-olds.)

The Spelling Retardates exhibit a difference of at least two years between chronological age and spelling age (Schonell's Graded Spelling Test A). In addition, the reading quotient calculated from the mental age derived from the WISC Full Scale IQ and reading age was 80 or less. The limitations and unreliability of reading quotients so derived are recognized but these did give a useful indication of the degree of reading backwardness. While the major problem in this group was spelling some degree of reading difficulty was also present but in every case less than that occurring in the first group.

27

Specific Dyslexia

Selection was carried out by a research assistant on the criteria described above. Neither the physicians nor the psychologists were aware when examining the children whether they would or would not be included in the experimental groups. The criteria for selection were applied in the following order: age, IQ, school factors of absence and change of school, severe emotional disturbance, physical status and degree of reading and spelling retardation. Excluded on such grounds were 155 boys. In a further 18 the data obtained were too incomplete for inclusion. This left 98 boys aged 8 years to 12 years 11 months who gave evidence of quite specific reading and spelling difficulties, 56 Reading Retardates and 42 Spelling Retardates. The distribution of the reasons for exclusion is tabulated below. While these as reported are mutually exclusive, in individual cases this was not necessarily so. The fact that the Centre was established to investigate the problems of children of at least average intelligence and who were physically normal meant that very few of those assessed were excluded on the grounds of too low IQ, or physical abnormality.

Table 1

Distribution of Primary Reasons for Omission from Experimental Groups

	Type of School		
Reason	*State (95)*	*Private (78)*	*Total (173)*
Age: 13 years +	6·3%	5·1%	5·8%
Less than 8 years	21·1%	21·8%	21·4%
IQ too low	8·4%	5·1%	7·0%
School factors	7·4%	7·7%	7·5%
Emotional disturbance	24·2%	15·4%	20·2%
Physically not normal	6·3%	2·6%	4·6%
Not retarded	16·8%	30·8%	23·1%
Incomplete information	9·5%	11·5%	10·4%
Total percentage	100	100	100

Of the 271 boys from whom the sample was selected, 154 attended State schools and 117 private schools. Of the 98 dyslexic boys selected, 59 came from State schools and 39 from private schools, this being approximately the same proportion as found in the total 271 cases. Of the 56 Reading Retardates, 33 attended State and 23 private schools. Of the 42 Spelling Retardates, 26 attended a State school and 16 a private school. The distribution of State and private schools in each group is similar, so that this sample provides no evidence that boys in private schools are more liable to specific reading or specific spelling problems than boys attending State schools.

Two points of interest emerged. Among those excluded on the grounds of emotional disturbance, the proportion of boys from State schools was greater than that from independent schools. Insufficient retardation as a reason for exclusion was more frequent among independent school boys than among State school boys and, because of the order in which the criteria were applied, none of these boys was deemed to be severely emotionally disturbed.

Controls
The data obtained from the dyslexic boys are assessed by comparison with those obtained from two groups of boys unselected for reading or spelling ability. The majority of children examined at the Centre come from the upper socio-economic classes. In order to attempt to control this bias, schools serving predominantly middle-class areas[1] were sought for the selection of the control groups. The private school controls came from two preparatory schools in London and the State school controls came from a primary and a comprehensive secondary school in south-west London. Two groups of boys were selected to match each experimental group on age allowing a difference of two months, and type of school, State or private. Since children came to the Centre from almost every part of England, it was impossible to match on individual schools. The groups were not matched for IQ, except in so far as similar lower limits relating to Full Scale IQ and Verbal IQ were applied.

With parental permission, the boys were examined at school during school hours. In each school a quiet room where testing could be carried out without interruption was put at the disposal of the examiners.

Age. The chronological age distributions, means and standard deviations are given in Table 2. The mean age of the Reading Retardates is approximately 8 months higher than that of the Spelling Retardates.

Table 2

Distribution of Age · Reading Retardates, Spelling Retardates and two Control Groups

Age	Reading Retardates	Control 1	Spelling Retardates	Control 2
8 to 8 yrs 11 mths	9	8	12	12
9 to 9 yrs 11 mths	11	12	9	12
10 to 10 yrs 11 mths	16	16	14	11
11 to 11 yrs 11 mths	11	8	6	5
12 to 12 yrs 11 mths	9	12	1	2
Mean age (months)	126·2	126·3	117·7	118·0
Standard deviation	15·44	15·68	13·63	13·63

Summary
Altogether 98 dyslexic boys were selected from 271 boys examined at the Word Blind Centre. All were of at least average intelligence, Full Scale IQ on the WISC being not less than 90 and in no case was Verbal IQ less than 85. They were of normal physical status and gave no evidence of gross neurological abnormality. They were judged to be emotionally stable and had had normal educational opportunities. They were assigned to one of two groups. Each of the 56 boys in the first group, Reading Retardates, has a reading age of 2 or more years below chronological age. Each of the 42 boys in the second group, Spelling Retardates, has a spelling age of 2 or more years below chronological age, and is also underfunctioning in reading, but less severely than any Reading Retardate.

Both groups were matched for age, sex and type of school with similar numbers of boys unselected for reading or spelling ability, of at least average intelligence and drawn from schools in predominantly middle-class areas.

[1] In north-east, central and south-west London.

5

Data Collection, Tests and Procedures

The data analysed in this study were obtained from parents, from schools and from a medical and psychological examination. Where possible obstetric reports were obtained from hospitals.

Information from Parents

The parents of all 196 boys were asked to complete a Family Information Questionnaire (see Appendix 2). This was sent to the parents so that they could answer the questions at leisure and with maximum accuracy. The questions were structured, pre-coded and in most cases alternative answers were offered. They related to details of the child's family, father's occupation, parents' ages, whether or not mother had worked and was working, other mother/child separations, perinatal history, developmental history, illnesses, behavioural problems and the presence of reading, spelling and speech difficulties and atypical laterality patterns in parents and siblings. Where relevant, as in questions relating to developmental history and illnesses, parents were encouraged to write "can't remember" rather than guess. The Family Information form was not returned by the parents of two boys, in the control group of the Spelling Retardates. The physicians and psychologists interviewed one or both parents spending at least an hour, and often longer. Some perinatal information was already recorded on the Family Information Questionnaire received before the children were examined. The physician checked this information and where necessary obtained further information. The psychologist obtained a history of inter-family relationships and of the behaviour of the child at home and at school. The resulting information considered in conjunction with the child's behaviour, attitudes and adjustment during the psychological examination was used as the basis of judgement as to whether the child was or was not emotionally maladjusted.

The parents of the boys in the control groups were not interviewed.

Information from Schools

A questionnaire and the Bristol Social Adjustment Guide (The Child in School) were sent to each child's school (see Appendix 2). The purpose of the former was to assist the Centre's staff in determining the extent to which a child was handicapped in school by his reading and/or spelling difficulty

30

and to obtain information about the specificity of the reading difficulty prior to our agreeing to carry out assessment at the Centre. Information from this questionnaire relating to attendance, parental interest in progress and behaviour and the school's estimate of intelligence on a five-point scale was used in this study.

The total score on the Bristol Social Adjustment Guide was one of the criteria in selecting the experimental groups and this therefore affects the interpretation of the analysis of the scores obtained from the Guide.

Medical Examination

All the boys were given a full general medical and neurological examination by the Honorary Medical Adviser to the Centre, Dr A. White Franklin, except for 14 of the Reading and Spelling Retardates who were examined by Dr Macdonald Critchley, Consulting Physician, National Hospital for Nervous Diseases, London. Only those whose physical condition was rated as normal and who gave no evidence of a grossly abnormal neurological condition were included in the experimental groups.

Psychological Examination

Psychological tests were carried out by the Centre's psychologists. When, as happened occasionally, the WISC had been recently administered, usually by an educational psychologist attached to a Local Education Authority, this test was not repeated. The subtest scaled scores as well as Verbal IQ, Performance IQ and Full Scale IQ were requested and recorded. To speed up the programme, two additional appointments were made. Both were graduates in psychology and were trained at the Centre in the use of the necessary tests given by them, which did not include tests of intelligence, reading or articulation

Tests

The choice of specific tests was determined by a number of considerations. The Centre's primary purpose has been the collection of data in order to identify those features characteristically associated with a specific reading and/or spelling disability. Since it is postulated that specific dyslexia is constitutionally determined and frequently associated with other developmental anomalies, tests exploring areas of psychological function which are dependent as much upon neurological organization and maturation as upon environmental opportunity are of particular theoretical interest. Environmental conditions may produce deficits due to a lack of opportunity to develop certain skills, but here the Centre's largely middle-class sample was an advantage in so far as cultural and linguistic deprivation was unlikely to be a major cause of any deficit.

The assessment procedures had to subserve two objectives. The first was to established the presence, severity, nature and cause of the learning difficulty. The second, equally important, was to indicate the teaching method appropriate to each child's difficulties. Tests were included to ascertain the presence or absence of skills upon which the normal acquisition of reading and spelling are thought to depend. The specifically weak areas in which training was needed as well as those areas in which the child was functioning most effectively had to be identified. An objective assessment could best be made by comparing a child's performance with standards already established as normal. The majority of tests were, therefore, those for which norms were available.

The tests had to be valid for the age range of the children included in this study. As the developmental anomalies found in dyslexic children are commoner among younger children and often absent among older ones (Critchley, 1964), the tests had to be sensitive to the expected improvement in performance with increasing age.

Lastly there was the limiting time factor and the effect on the child of prolonged testing. As it was, the battery selected required two sessions each lasting about two hours and this was felt to be quite long enough for any child.

The following tests were administered individually to all Reading and Spelling Retardates and also to the control groups, except that with the controls the Spelling Test was administered where possible to small groups of not more than four. When this was done, the children were placed sufficiently far apart to prevent copying.

(1) *Wechsler Intelligence Scale for Children (WISC)*. The WISC consists of two subscales, one of which measures the subject's verbal ability while the other measures his non-verbal or performance ability. Each subscale has six subtests. Three scores are derived, usually from the scaled scores of five verbal and five performance subtests, a Verbal IQ, a Performance IQ and a Full Scale IQ. The subtests which Wechsler (1949) recommends for the computation of the IQs are Information, Comprehension, Arithmetic, Similarities, Vocabulary (Verbal), Picture Completion, Picture Arrangement, Block Design, Object Assembly, Coding or Mazes (Performance). The first ten are ordinarily given and these were administered in this investigation. Digit Span, a supplementary Verbal subtest, was also given but was not included in computing the Verbal IQ. As Digit Span is seldom given in routine practice the Verbal IQs obtained without it in this study can more readily be compared with those obtained in normal practice.

(2) *Reading Tests*. A prose reading test and a word reading test were used to reveal different aspects of a child's reading ability. The prose reading test enables the examiner to observe whether or not children make intelligent use of contextual clues and the extent to which use is made of their sometimes considerable speaking vocabulary. The word reading type of test in which a list of words is presented without any contextual clue reveals the child's ability to recognize whole words automatically and his ability to analyse phonically and to synthesize words not immediately recognized.

(a) *The Neale Analysis of Reading Ability, Form A*. This is a series of prose passages each in the form of a short story. The test is timed and after each passage has been read aloud, set questions are asked and the responses noted. The test yields three scores relating to rate of reading, accuracy and comprehension. The system of scoring enables the examiner to note the type of errors made by a child. This test is of limited value at both ends of the scale, particularly the lower end. It provides insufficient material to assess the ability of children who have very little reading skill. The Accuracy of Reading ages range from 5 years 8 months to 13 years, the Rate of Reading ages from 6 years 6 months to 13 years and the Comprehension of Reading ages from 6 years 3 months to 13 years.

(*b*) *Schonell's Graded Word Reading Test.* This test has a reading age range from 5 to 15 years. At each year level there are ten words phonically both regular and irregular. Since there is no time limit the child has ample opportunity to use his mechanical word reading ability to the full. A single reading age is calculated.

(3) *Schonell's Graded Spelling Test A.* The spelling age range is from 5 to 15 years with ten words at each year level. The first ten are regular three-letter words but thereafter words phonically both regular and irregular are included.

(4) *Auditory Discrimination.* The ability to perceive fine differences of sounds increases with age, but by 8 years of age children should be able to discriminate accurately all speech sounds (Templin, 1957). Faulty sound discrimination could lead to some confusion in learning to associate a sound with its symbol.

Wepman's Test of Auditory Discrimination Form A was used. The test consists of forty pairs of words, each of thirty pairs differing with regard to only one phoneme. The child is seated with his back to the examiner so that no cue is obtained from the movements of the examiner's mouth when enunciating the words. Fine discrimination of sound is involved. A difficulty in identifying similar and different sounds could be due to a hearing loss. Children who made five or more errors were referred for audiological examination and those in whom a hearing loss was ascertained were excluded from the experimental groups.

(5) *Articulation.* Permission was obtained to use an Articulation Attainment Test devised for use by speech therapists by Miss Catherine Renfrew, Senior Speech Therapist, Churchill Hospital, Oxford. The test material comprises largely pictures of objects very familiar to young children which the child is asked to name. The pronunciation of one hundred phonemes, vowels and consonants, both single and in blends, is noted. The test was standardized on young children from 3 years 2 months to 6 years 1 month. While theoretically children of 7 years or more should achieve the maximum score of 100 on the test, some allowance was desirable for carelessness and local deviations, for example, "th" is pronounced as "f" in some parts of London. On Miss Renfrew's advice, scores of 97 to 100 inclusive were regarded as normal. Scores of 94 to 96 indicated poor articulation, of 90 to 93 mildly defective, of 85 to 89 moderately defective and of 84 or under severely defective articulation.

(6) *Sound Blending.* The ability to blend a sequence of sounds into meaningful whole words is essential in learning to read and involves a number of skills. The sounds themselves must be accurately heard, the sequence of sounds perceived, retained and reproduced in correct order and blended into a whole word.

The test was adapted from Monroe's Phoneme Blending Test (1932). It consisted of twenty monosyllabic words, five each of two, three, four and five letters, e.g. i-t, f-r-o-s-t. The latter sounds are enunciated at one-second intervals, being pronounced without distortion and as nearly as possible as pronounced in the word. The subject repeats these and attempts to blend them into whole words, as he might do in the reading situation.

(7) *Visual Retention.* Visuo-perceptual and visuo-spatial function are explored in the performance subtests of the WISC. In reading, whole word

recognition involves the recognition of visual patterns perceived previously. In writing, particularly words which are phonically irregular, the retention and reproduction of visually perceived patterns is involved. The ability to remember and reproduce visually presented forms was explored with Benton's Visual Retention Test, Form C. This was given as described for Administration A, that is, under conditions of immediate recall. All ten cards were used. Since the subject is required to draw the shapes he has been shown, it is essentially a visuo-motor task.

(8) *Motor Proficiency*. All the boys in the experimental groups were normal on physical examination with no evidence of spasticity, or gross defect in motor power, muscle tone or co-ordination. Fine motor control and co-ordination required further assessment since minor degrees of clumsiness and of poor co-ordination have been described in some dyslexic children. The Oseretsky Test of Motor Ability provides an objective measure but has not been validated. It takes a considerable time to administer fully. Bannatyne had devised at the Centre a shortened form of the Oseretsky Scale which was used until, in the summer of 1967, we could obtain the Test for Motor Proficiency, a version of the Oseretsky, modified and revised by Stott (1966) and his colleagues. There are five separate sections for each age level from 4 years 6 months to 16 years: Balance, Upper Limb Co-ordination, Manual Dexterity, Whole Body Co-ordination and Simultaneous Movement. For most items, each side of the body is separately tested. Procedures for administration and scoring are clearly described in the Manual. Although the validation of this Test of Motor Proficiency has not been completed nevertheless it was found to provide a most useful objective measure.

(9) *Right/Left Discrimination*. This is frequently reported as being associated with specific dyslexia. Hermann (1959) has postulated that directional confusion is one of the basic factors in congenital word-blindness,

The test of right-left discrimination used was described by Swanson and Benton (1955). It consists of twenty items and the instructions are given verbally, for example, "Show me your left hand." Poor performance could be due to confusion in naming "right" as "left," as well as to a directional confusion. If a child consistently interpreted "right" as "left" this verbal labelling confusion was ignored in scoring. Some of the instructions are lengthy and difficult for some children to remember. In such cases the instructions were repeated so that every effort was made to exclude difficulties other than the directional ones.

(10) *Laterality*. Atypical patterns of laterality, left-handedness and more particularly ambilaterality or mixed-handedness, cross-laterality, that is, lack of correspondence between the dominant hand and eye, are claimed to be especially common among dyslexic children. Hand dominance may be influenced by social pressures either directly or indirectly, whereas the preferential use of one foot is less likely to be so influenced. Because the neural pathways from upper and lower limbs to the cerebrum are similar in that those from the right side cross to the left cerebral hemisphere and those from the left side to the right hemisphere, both handedness and footedness are more likely to be related to cerebral dominance than eyedness, since the bundles of neural fibres from each eye divide and pass to both hemispheres. Hand preference was evaluated by noting the hand used for writing and the degree of unilateral dominance was assessed by Harris's Test of Simultaneous

Writing (1958). With a pencil in each hand, the subject is asked to write, as fast as possible, the numbers 1 to 12 in two vertical columns. The criteria for scoring in terms of strong right, moderate right, ambilateral, moderate left and strong left laid down by Harris were followed. Eye preference was assessed by two tasks described by Clark (1957). In the first, the child was required to look through a cone-shaped object. This was wide enough at one end to go over both eyes but tapered at the other end to an aperture about one inch wide. The child who believed he was viewing with both eyes could in fact view with one eye only. For the second task a toy kaleidoscope replaced the cylinder but essentially the activity was similar in that the kaleidoscope was held to one eye.

Footedness was also assessed in two situations, by asking the subjects to kick a ball and to hop on one foot.

From the information obtained on writing hand, eyedness and footedness, the incidence of cross laterality, of hand and foot correspondence and of hand, eye and foot concordance was calculated.

(11) *Finger Differentiation.* Of the three tests of Finger Differentiation devised for children and described by Kinsbourne and Warrington (1963 *a*), two were used in this study. These were the One or Two Fingers and the In-Between Fingers Tests. They were administered and scored according to Clarke's instructions (unpublished) since percentile scores had been calculated by Clarke on 212 boys between the ages of 6 years to 10½ years +. Both are essentially neurological tests.

The One or Two Fingers test requires the subject to say whether, with vision excluded, one or two fingers are being touched by the examiner.

In the In-Between Fingers Test, two fingers are touched and the subject required to say how many fingers lie between those touched, again with vision excluded.

Summary

Information obtained from the parents included details of developmental history, illnesses, behavioural problems, mother/child separations, and the presence of reading, spelling and speech difficulty and of left-handedness in the child's immediate family. From each boy's school details of school attendance, parental interest and an estimate of intelligence on a five-point scale were requested. The schools were also asked to complete the Bristol Social Adjustment Guide (The Child in School).

All boys were examined medically. Obstetric reports for those born in hospital were requested. Tests administered by a psychologist included the Wechsler Intelligence Scale for Children, Neale's Analysis of Reading Ability, Schonell's Graded Word Reading Test, Schonell's Spelling Test, Wepman's Test of Auditory Discrimination, Renfrew's Articulation Attainment Test, a test of Phoneme Blending (Sound Blending), Benton's Right/Left Discrimination Test, Stott's Test of Motor Proficiency or a shortened form of the Oseretsky Test of Motor Ability, Benton's Visual Retention Test, two tests of Finger Differentiation and tests of hand, eye and foot preference.

6

Home, School and Behaviour

Environmental conditions, particularly those relating to home and school, are of obvious importance in any study of children with reading difficulties. Do conditions at home favour or discourage the development of reading skills? Early mother/child separations can lead to emotional problems, one of the consequences of which can be a failure to learn to read. Socio-cultural deprivation is known to be a major factor in the general development of children and to contribute to backwardness in reading. Parental interest, or rather lack of interest, in their children's achievement has been shown to be associated with reading retardation (Davis and Kent, 1955). How far have such factors contributed to the reading difficulties of the boys in this sample?

To find reading and writing difficult is frustrating enough. Is there likely to be a further frustration because the boys are placed in classes or schools where they are unlikely to be given the opportunity to develop other talents, including those of an academic nature?

It was clearly of interest to find out how many boys had received some sort of extra help at school. This would give some indication of the extent to which these problems were recognized, even if their nature were not appreciated. Details of the kind of help given are also reported.

Finally this chapter contains comments made by parents and teachers on behaviour at home and at school. A child's behaviour at home and his behaviour at school may be very different, especially if different attitudes are taken by his parents and by his teachers. This sample of dyslexic boys was selected to exclude those with emotional problems severe enough to be a main cause of the difficulty, but the emotions of an intelligent child who experiences a specific difficulty in learning to read and to write and who fails miserably year after year are almost certain to be disturbed in some way; so too are those of his parents.

Tests of statistical significance were carried out on socio-economic status, parents' ages, birth order, family order, the number of working mothers and other mother/child separations. Otherwise the data reported in this chapter are purely descriptive.[1]

---

[1] The technique of Analysis of Variance was used in the comparison of mean scores. In each analysis account was taken of socio-economic class. Where the data are categorized the Chi-square test was employed. Only p values less than 0.05 are regarded as significant.

Home

Information was obtained from the parents relating to father's occupation, parental ages, adoption, the birth order of each child in relation to the natural mother, the position of the child in relation to the family with which he lived, whether or not mother had worked during the first four years of the child's life, whether mother was working at the time of the examination and other mother/child separations.

Socio-economic status

From father's occupation, socio-economic status was determined according to the classification provided by the Registrar-General (1960). The third category — Category III, Skilled Occupations — was divided into two groups separating non-manual workers from skilled manual workers.

Table 3
Social Class Based on Occupation of Father

	Reading Retardates	Control 1	Spelling Retardates	Control 2
Class I	14	14	13	12
Class II	23	29	25	15
Class III Non-manual	6	4	1	4
Class III Skilled-manual	10	7	2	6
Class IV	3	2	1	2
Class V	0	0	0	1
Total number	56	56	42	40
Chi-square 1 d.f.	$p > 0.05$		$p > 0.05$	

The majority of boys in both dyslexic groups belong to Classes I and II; this reflects the very biased socio-economic background of the children examined at the Centre. A deliberate attempt was made to find controls from backgrounds similar to those of the dyslexic children by selecting them from schools in middle-class areas. While the distribution of classes is very similar in the case of the Reading Retardates and their controls, there is a slightly higher number of boys among the Spelling Retardates from the upper two classes than among their controls. No significant differences were found.

Birth and Family Order

Seven boys were adopted, of whom 6 were dyslexic (3 Reading and 3 Spelling Retardates). The birth order of 6 of these boys and of 3 boys in the control groups was unknown. Almost half of the boys in each control group and the Spelling Retardates were first born but only approximately one-quarter of the Reading Retardates. Only 8 boys were fifth-born or later (4 Reading Retardates, 2 Control 1, 1 Spelling Retardate and 1 Control 2). No significant differences in birth order distribution were found.

While the order of the child, including the adopted boys, within the family revealed no differences of distribution between the Spelling Retardates and Control 2, the value of Chi-square for Reading Retardates and Control 1 was just below the 5 per cent level of significance.

Table 4
Birth and Family Order

	Reading Retardates	Control 1	Spelling Retardates	Control 2
Birth Order				
1st	14	26	18	20
2nd–4th	35	27	21	18
5th +	4	2	2	1
Total number	53	55	41	39
Chi-square 2 d.f.	$p > 0.05$		$p > 0.05$	
Order within family				
1st	13	25	18	20
2nd–4th	39	29	22	19
5th +	4	2	2	1
Total number	56	56	42	40
Chi-square 2 d.f.	$p > 0.05$		$p > 0.05$	

The number of single-child families does not explain the tendency for fewer Reading Retardates to be first born or the first child within the family. In each group, very few boys, either 4 or 5, were only children. Excluding these, approximately one-third of the Spelling Retardates, Control 1 and Control 2 were eldest children (33 per cent, 36 per cent and 37 per cent respectively). Only 16 per cent of the Reading Retardates were eldest children. Similar findings are reported in the Isle of Wight Survey, 20 per cent of 86 retarded readers and 34 per cent of 144 Controls being eldest children (Rutter, Tizard and Whitmore, 1970). Linguistic skills tend to be better developed at an early age in only or first-born children (Davis, 1937). While the ordinal position in the family is of no significance among the Spelling Retardates, the possibility that this may be a contributory factor in some severely retarded readers cannot be overlooked.

Parental Age at Birth of Child
Parental ages and also the difference between father's and mother's ages were calculated for each socio-economic class. The mean maternal age in each group ranged from 29·2 years to 30·7 years and the mean paternal age from 32·4 years to 33·9 years.

No significant differences were found between the groups in mother's or father's ages or in the differences between their ages (Appendix 1, Table 1).

Mothers who Worked

A minority of mothers in all groups had at some time worked during the first four years of each boy's life, about a third of these full-time. A comparison of the number of mothers working, either full- or part-time between each dyslexic group and its control revealed no significant differences.

At the time of examination, working mothers were more numerous but still a minority. Less than a third of these worked full-time. The differences between groups were negligible.

Table 5
Boys Whose Mothers Worked

	Reading Retardates	Control 1	Spelling Retardates	Control 2
During First 4 Years				
Not working	41	44	32	31
Full-time work	3 } 15	3 } 12	2 } 7	3 } 9
Part-time work	12	9	5	6
Total number	56	56	39	40
Chi-square 1 d.f.	$p > 0.05$		$p > 0.05$	
At The Time of Examination				
Not working	33	35	28	21
Full-time work	6 } 21	6 } 18	1 } 12	2 } 18
Part-time work	15	12	11	16
Total number	54	53	40	39
Chi-square 1 d.f.	$p > 0.05$		$p > 0.05$	

Other Mother/Child Separations

Short periods of separation during a boy's first four years occurred in approximately half of the total number of subjects in each group. These were separations due mainly to hospitalization of mother (illness, new baby) and/ or child, holidays or business. No differences were found between the groups, with regard to the numbers of boys who had or had not experienced such separations (Appendix 1, Table 2).

Summary

No significant differences were found between each dyslexic group and its respective control with regard to socio-economic class (based on father's occupation), mother's age, father's age or the difference between parents' ages, birth order, ordinal position in the family, though fewer Reading Retardates were eldest children (not statistically significant), the number of mothers who had worked during the first four years of the subjects' lives or at the time of examination, or the number of boys separated from mother during the first four years for reasons other than work.

School
The data reported in this section were obtained from parents and from the boys' schools. Information about the type of school attended at the time of examination and about the number of schools previously attended was obtained from parents. Both parents and schools were asked for details of extra tuition or help given at or outside school. Parents' reports have been used here, supplemented where necessary by information from schools. Teachers provided the data on school attendance and also on parental interest in the boys' progress and behaviour.

Type of School Attended
In each group of retardates, the proportion of boys attending a private school is considerable and no doubt reflects the socio-economic bias of this sample. However, many boys had been removed by their parents from state to private schools on account of their reading and writing difficulties in the hope that smaller classes would enable teachers to give more help. On the other hand, many children from private schools were referred to the Centre because there was no provision for helping them.

Table 6
Type of School Attended at the Time of Examination

	Reading Retardates	Control 1	Spelling Retardates	Control 2
State School: junior	24	23	25	24
secondary	9	10	1	2
	33	33	26	26
Private School	23	23	16	16
Total number	56	56	42	42

Junior school boys of at least average intelligence could not be found to match for age 2 junior school dyslexics (1 Reading and 1 Spelling Retardate).

The secondary schools attended by the dyslexic boys were either secondary modern (7 boys) or comprehensive (3 boys). None attended a grammar school, although 3 and possibly 4 of the 7 at secondary modern schools, were of grammar school intellectual calibre with Verbal and Performance IQs of 142, 132; 128, 113; 119, 125; 120, 107.

Among the children examined and taught at the Centre were many who in spite of high intelligence had not been given a place at grammar school. Indeed it was difficult, if not impossible, to persuade many Head Teachers that intelligent children *were* intelligent. Our experience fully bears out the conclusion drawn in the Inner London Education Authority's Interim Report on their Literacy Survey (1969) that for the majority of Head Teachers general backwardness and backwardness in reading are functionally equivalent. It is perhaps little wonder that so many parents, if they can afford to do so, transfer their children from state to private schools in the hope of providing educational opportunities appropriate to their sometimes considerable talents in other fields. The concept of a *specific* learning disability affecting such basic skills as reading and writing appears to be very difficult for many Head

Teachers to understand, and when they do, they are reluctant to make special provisions for the intelligent backward reader which will enable him to develop fully his potential and talents in other areas.

Number of Schools Attended

The number of schools attended by a boy was one of the criteria in selecting the dyslexic boys. No boy was included if he had had more than three changes of school excluding normal transfers such as from infant to junior school. No restriction on the number of schools attended by the control-group boys was applied. Since the number of changes of school was a criterion of selection, no statistical test of significance is carried out. There is an excess of Reading Retardates who had experienced two or three changes of school.

Table 7
Number of Changes of School since age 5, Excluding Normal Transfers, e.g. Infant to Junior

Number of Changes of School	Reading Retardates	Control 1	Spelling Retardates	Control 2
0	14	22	12	17
1	23	22	21	17
2	15	3	6	3
3	4	3	3	1
4	0	2	0	2
5	0	2	0	1
6 or more	0	2	0	1
Total number	56	56	42	42

Ten boys, in the control groups combined, had changed schools more than three times. Since they were of very varying ages and IQ, Reading and Spelling Quotients based on mental age and reading and spelling ages are quoted to give some indication of whether or not they were reading and spelling at appropriate levels. Reading and Spelling quotients were 93, 91; 89, 90; 97, 99; 93, 100; 95, 89; 99, 97; 93, 82; 99, 101; 81, 69; 105, 110. Only 1 boy was experiencing serious reading and spelling difficulties. There is no evidence from this very small number to suggest that frequent changes of school alone give rise to reading and spelling difficulties. However, frequent changes of school are likely to be an added burden to the child who is failing for other reasons. But not unnaturally many parents who are concerned about a lack of progress will move a child from one school to another in an attempt to find more help. None the less, absence from school and changes of school did not loom as large factors in excluding children from this sample (see Table 1).

School Attendance

None of the dyslexic boys had been absent from school for considerable periods during their first two years at school, this being one of the criteria on

which selection was made. At the time of examination, information was
requested from schools, but was not in all cases supplied, regarding the
regularity or otherwise of attendance during the current year. Attendance was
recorded as regular, occasionally absent, frequently absent.

Frequent absence was reported in the case of only 1 boy (Control 1) and
occasional absence in 6 (4 Reading, 1 Spelling Retardate and 1 Control 1). All
others for whom information was obtained attended school regularly.
(Appendix 1, Table 3.)

Teachers' Estimates of Parental Interest
Teachers were asked whether parents were interested in their child's progress
and behaviour and to comment on how parental interest was shown. These
were open questions. The answers given and the terms in which they are
couched reflect the teachers' attitudes to the parents and to the children as
well as the attitudes of the parents. The first two questions on whether
interest in progress and in behaviour was shown were generally answered by
"yes," "very," "slightly" or in terms which could be categorized under the
headings "interested — unqualified," "slightly interested" or "very
interested."

The answers to the third question on how parental interest was shown,
were much more varied and not so easy to classify. Information was not
provided in many cases.

Table 8
Teachers' Comments on Parental Interest

	Reading Retardates	Control 1	Spelling Retardates	Control 2
Comments on Interest in Progress				
Not interested	0	0	0	0
Slightly interested	1	0	2	0
Interested — unqualified	27	39	22	27
Very interested	22	3	15	2
Unknown	6	14	3	13
Comments on Interest in Behaviour				
Not interested	0	0	1	0
Slightly interested	1	0	1	0
Interested — unqualified	32	35	25	26
Very interested	11	1	10	1
Unknown	12	20	5	15
How Interest was Shown				
Sometimes visits	3	14	3	8
Often visits	12	9	9	11
Co-operative	13	2	7	2
Concerned	5	0	1	0
Over-anxious	7	2	8	0
Lack of affection	0	0	1	0
Unknown	16	29	13	21
Total number	56	56	42	42

Teachers' estimates of parental interest in progress. All parents of either dyslexic or control boys were thought to be interested. Responses indicated that only slight interest was shown by the parents of three boys (1 Reading, 2 Spelling Retardates). All others about whom information was received, were said to be interested or very interested. The use of the adjective "very" was restricted almost entirely to the dyslexic boys. This is not surprising, since unless the parents had been considerably interested they would not have made the effort to bring their children to the Centre for examination. It is also possible however that the use of "very" reflected to some extent an increased awareness on the part of the teachers of the effect of parental interest on children who were experiencing learning difficulties.

Teachers' estimates of parental interest in behaviour. A pattern of responses fairly similar to that of the previous question was found. The parents of only 1 boy (Spelling Retardate) were thought to show no interest in behaviour and the parents of 2 (1 Reading, 1 Spelling Retardate) only slight interest. Fewer were "very" interested in behaviour than in progress, the majority of responses indicating simply that the parents were interested. But again there was a greater preponderance of "very" in relation to dyslexic boys and possibly for the same reasons which influenced responses to the previous question.

How parental interest was shown. Comments on how parental interest was shown probably reflected teachers' attitudes more than the two previous questions. Answers included comments on the frequency with which parents visited the school, on their willingness to co-operate, on their concern and over-anxiety, and one comment on lack of affection. Teachers thought that "concern" and "over anxiety" were shown more frequently by the parents of dyslexic boys. Parents of dyslexic boys were also noted more frequently as being "co-operative." Most teachers are very aware of the effect of parental concern and anxiety on a child who is handicapped in some way. Concern is a natural expression of parental feeling and it would probably be true to say that the parents of all the dyslexic boys were "concerned." When parents feel that all that might be done to help their children is not being done, they may appear over-anxious because of the considerable efforts that they make on behalf of their children. But under these circumstances, it is wrong to assume that parental anxiety is a cause of the reading difficulty. It is just as likely to be an effect of it.

Extra Tuition received by Dyslexics

The nature of any help received is described separately for State and for private schools since it is of interest to know whether the two systems of education provided similar facilities for helping this sample of children with reading and spelling difficulties. Some caution must be exercised in interpreting the findings reported, since the information obtained relates to treatment received in the past as well as the present, and since several children had transferred from State to private schools (transfers from private to State schools were very rare). No information was obtained about 2 Spelling Retardates, both attending State schools, so that the total number of Spelling Retardates attending State schools is 24 in the tables below. No help had been given either at school or from any Local Authority Service to 14 boys attending State schools (4 Reading and 10 Spelling Retardates), and to

14 boys at private schools (7 Reading and 7 Spelling Retardates). Parents
were paying privately for the tuition of 7 of these boys, 4 in State and
3 in private schools.

Table 9
The Percentage of Dyslexics to whom No Help or
Some Help had been given

	Reading Retardates		Spelling Retardates		
---	State	Private	State	Private	Total
Type of School	*State*	*Private*	*State*	*Private*	*Total*
No help given	12·1%	30·4%	41·7%	43·7%	29·2%
Some help given	87·9%	69·6%	58·3%	56·3%	70·8%
Total number	33	23	24	16	96

Some help had been organized for 45 of the Reading Retardates (80·4 per
cent) and for 23 Spelling Retardates (57·5 per cent). While most of the boys
with severe specific reading difficulties had been given help of some kind,
almost 20 per cent had received none.

More than half of the Spelling Retardates had received extra tuition. While
not severely retarded in reading when examined at the Centre they were still
underfunctioning to a quite marked degree and were being educationally
handicapped by their difficulties in expressing themselves on paper. As a
group they were highly intelligent (mean Full Scale WISC 119) but all had
found learning to read difficult. They appeared, unlike the severely retarded
readers, to have overcome their difficulties although this was not the case. All
were in need of remedial teaching but this was rarely available and 43 per cent
had received no help at all.

Extra tuition or special arrangements took many forms both within and
outside school. In the school, these included placement in special classes or
placement in special groups which were either withdrawn from the class for
short periods or remained within the classroom. Individual help was most
often given by a member of the school staff and very rarely by a visiting
remedial teacher. Outside school, help was given in remedial classes or Child
Guidance Clinics. In addition several parents were paying for privately
arranged individual tuition.

Special classes, as distinct from special groups, tend to be classes for
generally backward children who need long-term tuition geared to a slower
rate of learning. The placement of intelligent children with a specific learning
difficulty in such classes proved frustrating to them and gave rise to complaints from the children and from their parents. Many boys were acutely
aware that they were not being given the opportunity to learn about
"interesting things." So not only was there frustration from being unable to
read and write adequately, there was the further frustration from being denied
the opportunity to develop their talents in other areas.

Details of the type of help given, are to be found in Table 4, Appendix 1.
The only help received by 22 boys (13 Reading and 9 Spelling Retardates)
was from an assistant teacher, generally the class teacher. Fifteen boys (6 Reading
and 9 Spelling Retardates) had been put into a special class and a further
20 (17 Reading and 3 Spelling Retardates) into a special group. Only 15 boys

(14 Reading and 1 Spelling Retardate) had received help from a remedial teacher, 10 of these attending a remedial class and 5 receiving tuition from a visiting remedial teacher. Eight boys (5 Reading and 3 Spelling Retardates) had at some time attended a Child Guidance Clinic.

One-third of the boys had received more than one type of help, the "extra" source of help provided by the class teacher in most cases.

The parents of 17 of the 68 boys who had been helped at school or at a Local Authority class or clinic, were paying for additional private tuition. No boy receiving tuition from a visiting remedial teacher had had extra private tuition. The parents of 24 of the total 98 boys had paid for private tuition.

It appears from Table 9 that help was received by fewer severely dyslexic boys in private than in state schools. Even if the transfer to private schools because of lack of help in State schools accounts for part of this difference, it would seem that less help was given in private schools. The kind of help given differed little between the two types of school. The chief difference lay in attendance at remedial classes, these being organized by Local Authorities.

Considerable efforts had clearly been made to help most of the boys (80 per cent of the Reading and 57 per cent of the Spelling Retardates). But only 15 of the total 68, who had had help at some time, had received it in a recognized remedial situation. The majority had been given help within the school, in special classes, special groups and individually by school teachers. The inadequacy of facilities is shown by the fact that these boys still had severe reading and spelling difficulties. This is no reflection on the teachers who had given unstintingly of their time and effort. Teachers have the wish to help but lack the knowledge. This is amply shown by the great number of requests received at the Word Blind Centre from teachers, mostly from the State schools, to visit and to learn what to do.

Failure to recognize the peculiar nature of these boys' difficulties could be another reason for the failure of tuition. The child with specific dyslexia has an inordinate difficulty in associating sounds with symbols, a difficulty un-related to the level of intelligence, and often associated with other develop-mental anomalies of the kind indicated in Chapter 2. Such children need the skills of experienced remedial teachers aware of each child's specific learning difficulty and having the knowledge and ability to plan teaching programmes to take these into account. To recognize the child's difficulty and to communicate it to the child and his parents is also very important. To learn that a child's difficulties do not stem from lack of effort or crass stupidity is often the first step towards regaining hope and the will to learn.

Behaviour

Parents were asked to record whether they had observed certain behavioural problems including nervousness, timidity, fears, naughtiness, jealousy or envy, temper tantrums, silent periods and nightmares. Space was provided in the Questionnaire (see Appendix 2) for any additional problems. The parents noted when such behaviour was exhibited, whether "at present," or "only in the past," or both "in the past and at present," or "never."

The Bristol Social Adjustment Guide (The Child at School) was completed by the teacher or Head Teacher and dealt with behaviour in school at about the time of the examination. The Guide consists of a large number of descrip-tions of behaviour and the teacher underlines those which are applicable to

Specific Dyslexia

the child. Descriptions of "normal" and of deviant behaviour are included. The latter are rearranged under the headings of specific types of deviant behaviour such as "Hostility towards adults," "Anxiety towards children," "Unforthcomingness," etc., on a Diagnostic Form.

Comments on a child's behaviour by parents and by school teachers reflect not only the child's behaviour but also the reaction of parent or of teacher to the child and to the particular mode of behaviour in question. What one parent might regard as a problem, another may not. Thus some parents in underlining "Never" added the comment "not more than usual." The conclusions which can be drawn from the findings reported below are limited by the exclusion from this sample of dyslexic boys of those deemed to be severely emotionally disturbed. The total score on the Bristol Social Adjustment Guide (BSAG) was one criterion of emotional disturbance. No boy with a score suggestive of emotional maladjustment (Stott, 1963) was included. Information from parental reports was not included among the selection criteria.

Parental Report of Behaviour.

The frequency with which the behavioural problems were noted is given below. No significant differences were found in any of the comparisons made, these being based on the number of boys who had never shown the features listed and the number who had at some time done so.

Table 10
Frequency of Behavioural Problems (Parental Report)

	Reading Retardates	Control 1	Spelling Retardates	Control 2
Jealousy or Envy				
Never	48	42	26	26
Past only	2	5	3	1
Present only	0	0	0	2
Past and present	5	8	11	8
Unknown	1	1	2	5
Temper Tantrums				
Never	33	37	25	25
Past only	9	9	3	7
Present only	2	2	0	1
Past and present	11	7	13	7
Unknown	1	1	1	2
Silent Periods				
Never	51	52	37	37
Past only	3	0	0	1
Present only	2	0	0	0
Past and present	0	3	2	2
Unknown	0	1	3	2
Nightmares				
Never	41	44	28	24
Past only	9	9	10	9
Present only	1	0	1	1
Past and present	4	2	1	5
Unknown	1	1	2	3

	Reading Retardates	Control 1	Spelling Retardates	Control 2
Nervousness				
Never	38	32	26	28
Past only	1	13	3	2
Present only	2	0	3	0
Past and present	14	9	9	10
Unknown	1	2	1	2
Timidity				
Never	38	41	26	28
Past only	5	5	3	4
Present only	0	1	2	0
Past and present	10	8	7	6
Unknown	3	1	4	4
Fearfulness				
Never	36	33	26	20
Past only	8	15	5	8
Present only	1	1	1	0
Past and present	9	6	7	8
Unknown	2	1	3	6
Naughtiness				
Never	43	37	25	24
Past only	2	6	2	3
Present only	1	0	2	0
Past and present	9	11	7	11
Unknown	1	2	6	4

Dyslexic boys were the only ones reported to be nervous, naughty or to have silent periods at the time of examination only, the number being very small (5, 3 and 2 respectively). Temper tantrums occurring both in the past and present are a little more frequently reported for dyslexic boys (11 Reading Retardates, 7 Control 1, 13 Spelling Retardates, and 7 Control 2).

A history of head-banging or rocking was reported in 4 boys (2 Reading, 1 Spelling Retardate and 1 Control 2). Sleepwalking, talking in sleep or insomnia were reported in 6 boys (3 Reading Retardates, 2 Control 1 and 1 Control 2) and nail-biting or thumb-suckling in 6 boys (3 Spelling Retardates and 3 Control 1). Only a history of head-banging or rocking, among these further problems volunteered by parents, was noted predominantly among the dyslexics but since the parents were not specifically asked whether there was such a history, there may have been other unreported cases. One child was reported to have had a nervous tic (Control 1).

The number of behavioural problems reported for each boy was calculated, the resulting scores ranging from 0 to 8. Some questions had not been answered in the questionnaires, but the total number of missing items was identical in the case of the Reading Retardates and Control 1. In Control 2, 27 items were unknown as against 22 for the Spelling Retardates. The dyslexic boys were not reported by their parents to have shown a greater number of behavioural problems than the Control boys. The parents of the dyslexic boys may have been loath to report deviant behaviour. However since more than two-thirds of the dyslexics could be classified as "stable" and none were "maladjusted" on teachers' reports, it is more probable that the parents' reports were reliable.

Table 11
The Distribution of the Number of Behavioural Problems
Reported for Individual Boys

	Reading Retardates	Control 1	Spelling Retardates	Control 2
No problem	11	15	7	8
1 or 2 problems	25	17	14	14
3 or 4 problems	13	13	13	12
5 or 6 problems	5	10	6	4
7 or 8 problems	2	1	1	2
Total number of boys	56	56	41	40

There is no difference in the distribution of those with no problem and those with some problem between either dyslexic group and its control. Nor is there any evidence that a greater number of problems were exhibited by the dyslexic boys.

Behaviour in School – Bristol Social Adjustment Guide
Since the total number of adverse responses on the Bristol Social Adjustment Guide (The Child in School) was one of the criteria for the selection of the dyslexic boys, no tests of statistical significance are carried out. Notwithstanding the exclusion of boys with a total score of 20 or more, suggestive of maladjustment, it is of interest to note the numbers of boys in this sample who might be regarded as stable or quasi-stable, score 0 to 9, or unsettled, score 10 to 19 (Stott, 1963) and to note any particular attitudes or response patterns which appear to occur more frequently among the dyslexics.

The mean total scores for the four groups were Reading Retardates 7·8, SD 5·34, Control 1 5·2, SD 7·09, Spelling Retardates 6·9, SD 5·65, Control 2 6·2, SD 5·89. Thus while Spelling Retardates and their controls present a very similar range of scores, the Reading Retardates as a group tend to exhibit a greater number of adjustment problems. This is further reflected in the greater number of "unsettled" boys, 30·4 per cent among the Reading Retardates, compared with 12·5 per cent among Control 1 boys. Of the Spelling Retardates 21·4 per cent were "unsettled" and a greater number, 23·8 per cent, of Control 2 boys.

Table 12
The Bristol Social Adjustment Guide (The Child in School):
Adjustment Category and Mean Total Score

	Reading Retardates	Control 1	Spelling Retardates	Control 2
Stable or quasi-stable (0–9)	69·6%	82·1%	78·6%	71·4%
Unsettled (10–19)	30·4%	12·5%	21·4%	23·8%
Maladjusted (20 and over)	0·0%	5·4%	0·0%	4·8%
Total Score				
Mean	7·8	5·2	6·9	6·2
SD	5·34	7·09	5·65	5·89
Total number	56	56	42	42

Table 13
The Bristol Social Adjustment Guide: Presence and
Degree of Specific Attitudes and Responses

	Reading Retardates	Control 1	Spelling Retardates	Control 2
Unforthcomingness				
None or slight	51	53	40	38
Some	5	3	2	4
Strong	0	0	0	0
Depression				
None or slight	44	46	32	35
Some	12	10	10	7
Strong	0	0	0	0
Withdrawal				
None or slight	53	55	42	40
Some	3	1	0	2
Strong	0	0	0	0
Anxiety Towards Adults				
None or slight	47	53	38	36
Some	9	3	4	5
Strong	0	0	0	1
Hostility Towards Adults				
None or slight	50	50	37	37
Some	6	3	5	4
Strong	0	3	0	1
Unconcern				
None or slight	44	52	38	38
Some	12	3	4	4
Strong	0	1	0	0
Anxiety Towards Children				
None or slight	49	52	39	38
Some	7	4	3	4
Strong	0	0	0	0
Hostility Towards Children				
None or slight	50	51	37	40
Some	6	5	5	2
Strong	0	0	0	0
Restlessness				
None or slight	42	52	35	38
Some	14	4	7	4
Strong	0	0	0	0
Emotional Tension				
Mean Score	0·6	0·3	0·7	0·2
Total number	56	56	42	42

Why so many boys in Control 2 should exhibit "unsettledness" cannot be explained. These boys were selected from the same schools as the boys in Control 1 and there was no indication from parental reports of an excess of behavioural problems among them.

The presence and degree of the various types of deviant behaviour recorded on the Guide were determined by the criteria suggested by Stott. On these criteria no boy was severely withdrawn, unforthcoming, depressed or hostile to children nor did any reveal severe anxiety in relation to children. Severe anxiety towards adults was shown by only 1 boy (Control 2), severe hostility to adults by 4 (3 Control 1, 1 Control 2), severe unconcern by 1 (Control 1) and severe restlessness by 1 (Control 2). Some anxiety towards adults, hostility towards adults, unconcern, and restlessness were slightly more prevalent among the Reading Retardates than in any other group. There were more signs of emotional tension among both dyslexic groups.

Discussion

In the Isle of Wight Survey (Rutter, Tizard and Whitmore, 1970) questionnaires completed by parents and by teachers and a psychiatric interview were used to assess emotional and behavioural disturbance in children with a specific reading retardation. On both questionnaires these children obtained much higher scores than the control group, anti-social behaviour rather than neurotic disorder being more prevalent. No evidence was found in that study to support the view that emotional disturbance was a cause of the reading failure. Using what appeared to be arbitrary cut-off points, a greater number of specifically retarded readers obtained scores above the cut-off points on the teachers' than on the parents' questionnaires. In this study, teachers' assessments were used as one of the selecting criteria. Estimates of correspondence between parents' and teachers' assessments were not made but the number of boys reported by parents to be currently exhibiting behavioural problems was small and the number of problems no greater among the dyslexics than among the controls. However, almost a third of the Reading Retardates and approximately one-fifth of the Spelling Retardates were classifiable as "unsettled" on the teachers' assessment of current behaviour, compared with about one-eighth of Control 1. Discrepancies between parents' and teachers' reports could arise for a number of reasons but it is quite likely that in school, where the specific learning difficulty cannot be avoided, children exhibit behavioural difficulties which are not apparent at home.

7

Results of Psychological Tests and Developmental History

The tests administered by the psychologist are described in Chapter 5 and comprised those of intelligence, reading, spelling, articulation, auditory discrimination, sound blending, visual retention, right/left discrimination, finger localization, motor proficiency, handedness, eyedness and footedness. The form used to record results is reproduced in Appendix 2.

This chapter deals with the results of these tests. Since tests of speech (articulation) and motor proficiency are included, it seemed more relevant to report here information about the development of speech and motor function. The results are discussed in Chapter 9, together with the results of the physical examination to allow a composite and meaningful interpretation.[1]

Attainment in Reading

The Reading Age of all Reading Retardates was at least two years below chronological age. The Spelling Retardates were not so severely retarded in reading, none reading at a level of two or more years behind chronological age. The mean reading retardation in relation to mean chronological age (see Table 2) varies between 40 to 49 months in the case of the Reading Retardates and between 5 to 14 months in the Spelling Retardates.

In both control groups matched for age and type of school and from predominantly middle-class background, the majority of boys were reading far in advance of their chronological age. That the Reading Retardates were experiencing considerable difficulties is evident, but their difficulties become even more marked in comparison with the standards attained by the control groups, and the less backward Spelling Retardates were reading on an average, at a level about 2½ years below their controls. In such circumstances what appears to be a minor degree of retardation can cause concern to parents and to teachers and not least to the child himself.

Four of the 98 control boys, 4·1 per cent, were retarded in reading by more than 2 years (25 months, 27 months, 29 months and 39 months) in relation to chronological age.

---

[1] The technique of Analysis of Variance was used in the comparison of mean scores. In each analysis account was taken of socio-economic class. Where the data are categorized, the Chi-square test was employed. Only p values less than 0·05 are regarded as significant.

Table 14
Reading and Spelling Ages (in Months): Reading Retardates
Spelling Retardates and two Control Groups

	Reading Retardates		Control 1		Spelling Retardates		Control 1	
	Mean	SD*	Mean	SD	Mean	SD	Mean	SD
Neale Analysis Of Reading Ability								
Accuracy	86·4	15·54	136·7	16·04	105·4	17·21	131·4	18·51
Rate	81·9	17·92	139·4	19·96	103·8	17·76	132·2	21·63
Comprehension	86·1	16·38	140·3	14·70	112·0	28·00	135·1	18·64
Schonell's Graded Word Reading Test	84·4	17·40	143·5	20·60	106·1	22·13	136·1	22·36
Schonell's Graded Spelling Test A	79·9	14·31	132·1	23·86	89·9	11·92	124·6	24·56
Total number	56		56		42		42	

*Standard Deviation.

Table 15
Retardation in Reading Accuracy in Relation to Chronological Age
Neale Analysis of Reading Ability

	Reading Retardates	Spelling Retardates	Total	Control 1	Control 2	Total
Not retarded	0	5	5	43	37	80
Retarded by						
1 to 11 months	0	13	13	11	3	14
12 to 23 months	0	24	24	0	0	0
24 to 35 months	24	0	24	1	2	3
36 to 47 months	20	0	20	1	0	1
48 to 59 months	6	0	6	0	0	0
60 to 71 months	5	0	5	0	0	0
72 to 83 months	1	0	1	0	0	0
Total number	56	42	98	56	42	98

Attainment in Spelling

The mean spelling ages are lower than the mean reading ages. While reading and spelling ages cannot be directly compared, since they are based on tests standardized on different populations, it is common for reading skills to be in advance of spelling among junior school children. In spelling as in reading, the mean attainment age for both control groups is above mean chronological age.

Table 16
Retardation in Spelling in Relation to Chronological Age
Schonell's Graded Spelling Test

	Reading Retardates	Spelling Retardates	Total	Control 1	Control 2	Total
Not retarded	0	0	0	35	29	64
Retarded by						
1 to 11 months	0	0	0	11	8	19
12 to 23 months	2	0	2	6	3	9
24 to 35 months	8	35	43	3	0	3
36 to 47 months	23	6	29	1	2	3
48 to 59 months	9	1	10	0	0	0
60 to 71 months	12	0	12	0	0	0
72 to 83 months	2	0	2	0	0	0
Total number	56	42	90	56	42	98

The spelling age of 34 of the 98 controls was below chronological age but only 6 boys were retarded by two or more years, of whom 4 were the backward readers referred to above. One of the remaining 2 was retarded in reading by 11 months and the other was reading in advance of his chronological age although spelling 38 months below it.

Reversals, Transposition of Letters and Bizarre Spelling
A proneness in writing to reverse letters, transpose letters within a word or to spell in a bizarre fashion where the written word bears little or no resemblance to the sound of a word, could not be reliably explored. Many of the Reading Retardates knew no or few letters and the younger Spelling Retardates were not much better, being able to write too few words to reveal these errors. Since levels of spelling varied, those whose spelling was at a higher level and who attempted a greater number of words would have had more opportunity to make these mistakes than those who could write only a few words. Two short dictated sentences[1] could not be attempted fully or even in part by many of the dyslexics. All of the control boys were able to write it, although not necessarily spelling each word correctly. Among the controls only one

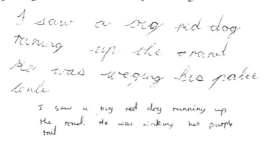

Fig. 1
Above: Dyslexic boy aged 12 years 8 months, IQ 107
Below: Control aged 12 years 10 months, IQ 111.

[1] I saw a big red dog running up the road.
He was wagging his purple tail.

reversal was made, b for d. Only 1 boy produced one letter transposition within a word and no boy wrote in a bizarre fashion. Some words were incorrectly spelled, but they were phonically written and there was no doubt, when reading the sentence, about the words a boy intended to write. Among the dyslexics letter reversals were made by 22 of the 65 who could produce the sentence. Only 8 transposed letters but 17 wrote words which could only be described as bizarre.

It is doubtful whether a proneness towards making these errors could be reliably ascertained in a single testing situation. A child's school exercise books will provide more information than his writing of a list of words or a sentence, particularly in a test situation where he is making more than usual effort.

Intelligence

Wechsler Intelligence Scale for Children (WISC)
All of the subtests were given with the exception of mazes. In calculating the Verbal IQ, Digital Span was omitted. The Analyses of Variance carried out on Full Scale IQ, Verbal IQ, Performance IQ and the subtests made allowance for socio-economic class. Three analyses were made for each item:
(*a*) Reading Retardates and Control 1; (*b*) Spelling Retardates and Control 2; and (*c*) to see whether the differences between Reading Retardates and their controls were significantly greater than the differences between Spelling Retardates and their controls, a significant difference indicating a dissimilarity between Reading and Spelling Retardates and no significant difference indicating a similarity.

Table 17
Wechsler Intelligence Scale for Children:
Intelligence Quotients

	Reading Retardates		Control 1		Spelling Retardates		Control 2	
	Mean	SD	Mean	SD	Mean	SD	Mean	SD
Full Scale IQ	107·1	8·95	120·0	11·97***	119·0	10·15	120·5	13·62
Verbal IQ	105·2	9·49	121·0	14·54***	117·3	10·40	120·5	12·23
Performance IQ	107·9	10·85	115·2	11·33**	117·7	11·10	116·4	15·12
Total number	56		56		42		42	

** Difference between means significant at 1% level.
*** Difference between means significant at 0·1% level.

Significant differences between the Reading Retardates and their controls are found in respect of Full Scale, Verbal and Performance IQ but not between the Spelling Retardates and their controls. On the three intelligence quotients the differences between Reading Retardates and their controls are significantly greater than the differences between the Spelling Retardates and their controls, indicating dissimilarity between the two groups of Retardates.

The mean intelligence quotients of both control groups are high, but not unexpectedly so, since the boys in these groups were selected from schools in predominantly middle-class areas. Both control groups show a higher verbal than performance mean IQ, which probably reflects the rich linguistic background of middle-class children. Although discrepancies between verbal and performance scores occurring in both directions have been described in children with reading difficulties (Kinsbourne and Warrington, 1963 b), more commonly reported is a greater preponderance of negative discrepancies with Verbal IQ lower than Performance IQ (Belmont and Birch, 1966; Warrington, 1967; Rutter, Tizard and Whitmore, 1970). Among the Reading Retardates, verbal scores were lower than performance scores in 37 cases but in only 15 of their controls ($p < 0.001$). Among the Spelling Retardates, a negative discrepancy occured in only 18 cases, less than half the total, as against 17 cases in their control group.

Table 18

Direction and Size of Discrepancy between Verbal and Performance IQ

	Reading Retardates	Control 1	Spelling Retardates	Control 2
Verbal greater than Performance				
No. of points				
1–9	6	15	17	11
10–19	9	16	4	8
20–29	3	7	1	4
30+	0	2	0	1
	18	40	22	24
Performance greater than Verbal				
No. of points				
1–9	18	6	9	13
10–19	17	6	7	4
20–29	2	1	2	0
30+	0	2	0	0
	37	15	18	17
No discrepancy	1	1	2	1
Total number	56	56	42	42

The mean of the difference between each boy's Verbal-Performance IQ was calculated for each group. The mean of Control 1 is higher than that of the Reading Retardates ($p < 0.001$) but the comparison between the Spelling Retardates and Control 2 just failed to reach a significant level. Differences between means reflected higher Verbal than Performance IQs among the controls as well as lower Verbal than Performance IQs among dyslexics. The difference between the Reading Retardates and Control 1 is not significantly greater than the difference between the Spelling Retardates and Control 2. Although their IQs are higher, the Spelling Retardates do not differ significantly from the Reading Retardates with regard to the extent of Verbal-Performance IQ discrepancy.

Discrepancies of 20 points or more were found in only 8 of the dyslexic boys (5 Reading Retardates and 3 Spelling Retardates) as against 17 of the control. But while such discrepancies among the dyslexics occurred equally in positive and negative directions, in only 3 of the controls was the discrepancy negative. All 3 of these boys were retarded in both reading and spelling, 2 seriously and one moderately. Among the 14 controls with large positive discrepancies 5 were backward in spelling to a marked degree in relation to IQ and in 2 of these reading was also poor.

While the Reading Retardates are not "dull" they may appear to be so by comparison with other boys at similar types of school and from similar backgrounds. This however cannot be said of the Spelling Retardates who were reading on average at a level approximately 2½ years below their control groups. It could be argued that middle-class boys of average intelligence are under pressure which would aggravate any initial difficulty in learning to read. However, this argument would not apply in all cases since Verbal, Performance and Full Scale IQs of 120 or more were found in 8, 10 and 7 boys respectively, and moreover it is doubtful whether the composite intelligence quotients are reliable indicators of intelligence when there are marked discrepancies between subtest scaled scores.

Subtests. The mean subtest scaled scores are given in Tables 19 and 20.

Three Reading and one Spelling Retardates had been given the WISC a short time before their examination at the Word Blind Centre and all or some

Table 19
WISC Subtest Scaled Scores: Reading Retardates and Control 1

	Reading Retardates			Control 1			Difference between Means
	No.	Mean	SD	No.	Mean	SD	p
Information	55	9·6	2·30	56	13·9	3·11	< 0·001
Comprehension	54	11·9	2·90	56	12·3	3·01	> 0·05
Arithmetic	53	8·8	2·88	56	12·7	3·31	< 0·001
Similarities	55	12·2	2·35	56	13·6	2·99	< 0·05
Vocabulary	53	11·8	1·85	56	14·2	2·72	< 0·001
Digit Span	53	8·3	2·27	56	11·6	3·08	< 0·001
Picture Completion	54	11·5	2·79	56	12·1	2·53	> 0·05
Picture Arrangement	55	10·6	2·48	56	11·2	2·70	> 0·05
Block Design	55	12·2	2·30	56	13·4	2·92	< 0·05
Object Assembly	55	11·5	2·66	56	12·1	2·08	> 0·05
Coding	55	9·5	2·45	56	12·2	2·28	< 0·001

Table 20
WISC Subtest Scaled Scores: Spelling Retardates and Control 2

	Spelling Retardates			Control 2			Difference between Means
	No.	Mean	SD	No.	Mean	SD	p
Information	41	12·1	2·20	42	13·5	2·61	< 0·01
Comprehension	41	12·9	2·67	42	12·2	2·41	> 0·05
Arithmetic	41	11·9	2·43	42	13·0	2·79	< 0·05
Similarities	41	13·6	2·68	42	13·7	2·63	> 0·05
Vocabulary	41	13·7	1·75	42	14·1	2·13	> 0·05
Digit Span	41	9·6	2·42	42	11·8	2·72	< 0·001
Picture Completion	41	13·1	3·39	42	12·7	3·15	> 0·05
Picture Arrangement	41	11·2	2·89	42	11·1	2·74	> 0·05
Block Design	41	14·5	2·58	42	13·6	3·13	> 0·05
Object Assembly	41	13·0	2·68	42	12·0	3·19	> 0·05
Coding	41	10·5	2·25	42	12·3	2·58	< 0·001

of the subtest scaled scores were not communicated. No significant differences were found between either of the dyslexic groups and their controls in respect of Comprehension, Picture Completion, Picture Arrangement and Object Assembly.

The scores of both dyslexic groups were significantly lower on Information, Arithmetic, Digit Span and Coding, all verbal subtests with the exception of Coding, which has a verbal component in that numbers are involved.

Only the Reading Retardates obtained significantly lower scores on Vocabulary, Similarities and Block Design, the last two significant at the 5 per cent level.

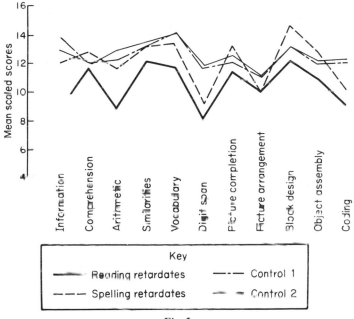

Fig. 2
Profiles of WISC mean subtest scaled scores:
Reading Retardates, Spelling Retardates, Control 1 and Control 2.

When differences between Reading Retardates and their controls were compared with differences between the Spelling Retardates and their controls, these were not significant with regard to Comprehension, Similarities, Digit Span, Picture Completion, Picture Arrangement, Object Assembly and Coding. Thus although the mean scores of the Reading Retardates were lower on these subtests than those of the Spelling Retardates, they were not so low as significantly to differentiate the Reading Retardates from the Spelling Retardates.

Significant differences between Reading and Spelling Retardates in relation to the control groups were obtained on Information, Arithmetic, Vocabulary and Block Design. Significant deficits on Information and Arithmetic were shown by both dyslexic groups, but were greater among the

Reading Retardates than among the Spelling Retardates. The Vocabulary and Block Design scores of the Spelling Retardates were not significantly lower than those of their control group so that these two subtests differentiate the Reading Retardates not only from their control group but also from the Spelling Retardates.

Internal inconsistency. An uneven profile on the WISC has been said to be typical of dyslexic children (Shedd, 1968). WISC profiles based on the mean subtest scaled scores for each of the four groups are illustrated in Fig. 2. The profiles of the control groups are almost identical and reveal a certain unevenness, the general pattern of which is reflected in the profiles of both groups of dyslexics. The unevenness in the latter is much more striking and throws doubt on the value of a composite intelligence quotient, particularly when Information, Arithmetic and Coding are included among the subtests.

Summary

The mean Full Scale, Verbal and Performance IQs of the Reading Retardates are significantly lower than those of their control group. The mean IQs of the Spelling Retardates are very similar to those of their controls and are certainly not lower. The mean Performance IQ is slightly higher in the Spelling Retardates.

The Verbal IQ is lower than the Performance IQ significantly more frequently only among the Reading Retardates. However, the mean difference between Verbal and Performance IQ is no greater among the Reading Retardates than among the Spelling Retardates. A discrepancy of 20 points or more between the Verbal and Performance IQ was found with equal frequency in positive and negative directions among the dyslexics whereas among the controls the Verbal IQ tended to be the higher.

Both dyslexic groups obtained significantly lower scores on Information, Arithmetic, Digit Span and Coding. The Reading Retardates were in addition poorer on Vocabulary, Similarities and Block Design.

A comparison of the differences between Reading Retardates and their control group and Spelling Retardates and their control group indicated that the two dyslexic groups did not differ significantly on Comprehension, Similarities, Digit Span, Picture Completion, Picture Arrangement, Object Assembly or Coding.

The two dyslexic groups do reveal significant differences with regard to Information, Arithmetic, Vocabulary, Block Design, and Full Scale, Verbal and Performance IQs. The difference between the dyslexic groups is one of degree rather than of different pattern and there are more similarities between them than differences. Apart from Coding it is the verbal subtests on which performance is poor.

Teachers' Estimates of Intelligence and WISC Intelligence Quotients

Estimates of intelligence on a five-point scale were made by 169 teachers and related to 89 dyslexics and 80 controls. The teachers were asked to rate the boys as "very bright," "bright," "average," "below average" and "limited." The questionnaire sent to schools included a space for entering an IQ if this were known. No intelligence test result was reported for any boy among the controls but the teachers of 31 dyslexic boys recorded an IQ resulting from a previously given group or individual intelligence test. Details of the WISC intelligence quotients for each category of the teachers' estimates are given in Table 5, Appendix 1, these being classified by private and State schools and by whether an IQ was or was not reported by the teachers.

If WISC IQs are regarded as reliable indicators of intellectual calibre, an assumption which cannot always be made, many boys, both dyslexic and control, were over-estimated as bright or very bright.

More striking, however, is the number of boys, again both dyslexic and control, who were estimated as of average or below average intelligence. There were 9 boys (6 dyslexic and 3 controls) with a Verbal and Performance IQ of 120 or more who were thought to be of not more than average intelligence. Rated as of "limited" intelligence were 3 dyslexic boys with a Verbal and Performance IQ of 96, 111; 116, 87; 118, 111 respectively. The one control boy so described had a Performance IQ of 111.

The lack of uniformity regarding knowledge of previous testing, the large number of schools involved with varying pupil intake, and academic standards will all affect the placement of individual children on a five-point scale. No conclusions can therefore be drawn..However, both over- and under-estimates of potential must have an effect on expectations and on the management of children.

Speech and Language

All the boys, dyslexic and control, were of European or American descent. Ten families were bilingual, only one of these being the family of a dyslexic child (Reading Retardate). The country in which the children were born was not recorded in 9 cases (4 dyslexics and 5 controls). The remaining 189 boys were born in an English-speaking country.

Early Speech and Language Development
Information was obtained from the parents about the age at which the boys used Mama/Dada, an additional four or five words, sentences of several words and the age at which pronunciation was clear to strangers. Often parents in all groups could not remember the relevant ages and were asked to record "Can't Remember." Several added the comment "average," "early" or "late." The frequency with which "Can't Remember" was recorded is not significant in any of the group comparisons. The parents were also asked to note whether they had observed articulatory defects and language difficulties. None recorded "Can't remember."

Speech Milestones
Mama/Dada tended to be spoken later by both Reading Retardates and Spelling Retardates in relation to their respective control groups, the mean ages being 11·0 months, 10·0 months, 11·4 months and 9·8 months for Reading Retardates, Control 1, Spelling Retardates and Control 2 respectively. However, the majority of children in all groups for whom information was available were using Mama/Dada by 14 months.

Both Reading and Spelling Retardates were slightly later in acquiring an additional four or five words, the mean ages being 17·3 months, 15·1 months 17·0 months and 13·8 months for Reading Retardates, Control 1, Spelling Retardates and Control 2 respectively.

Specific Dyslexia

Table 21
Speech Development — Words and Sentences

	Reading Retardates	Control 1	Spelling Retardates	Control 2
Age at which Mama/Dada spoken				
less than 12 months	57·1%	75·7%	53·6%	69·6%
12 to 14 months	21·4%	10·8%	21·4%	13·0%
15 months or later	21·4%	13·5%	25·0%	17·4%
Chi-square 2 d.f.		$p > 0.05$		$p > 0.05$
Mean age (months)	11·0	10·0	11·4	9·8
Number known	28	37	28	23
Number "Can't remember"	24	18	9	15
Number unknown	4	1	5	4
Age at which Additional 4 or 5 words spoken				
less than 15 months	34·6%	48·4%	37·0%	57·1%
15 to 23 months	34·6%	38·7%	51·8%	33·3%
24 months or later	30·8%	12·9%	11·1%	9·5%
Chi-square 2 d.f.		$p > 0.05$		$p > 0.05$
Mean age (months)	17·3	15·1	17·0	13·8
Number known	26	31	27	21
Number "Can't remember"	26	24	10	16
Number unknown	4	1	5	5
Age at which Sentences were used				
less than 18 months	7·7%	27·8%	14·3%	23·8%
18 to 29 months	53·8%	63·9%	57·1%	66·7%
30 months or later	38·5%	8·3%	28·6%	9·5%
Chi-square 2 d.f.		$p < 0.01$		$p > 0.05$
Mean age (months)	27·8	20·6**	26·5	21·2*
Number known	26	36	28	21
Number "Can't remember"	26	20	8	16
Number unknown	4	0	6	5

*Difference between means significant at 5% level.
**Difference between means significant at 1% level.

Percentages and means in this table and those following are based on the number of cases where information is available, i.e. "number known."

No significant differences are found until the boys reached the age at which sentences were used. The mean age for the Reading Retardates is 27·8 months and for their controls, 20·6 months ($p < 0.01$); for the Spelling Retardates it is 26·5 months and for their controls, 21·2 months ($p < 0.05$). More than one-third of the Reading Retardates and more than one-quarter of the Spelling Retardates were not using sentences till 30 months or later compared with less than a tenth of the boys in each control group.

Intelligibility, Articulation and Language
The age at which the boys' pronunciation was clear to strangers was reported in years. Among the control boys, only 2, 1 in each control group, were not speaking clearly before the age of 4 years, compared with 14 Reading Retardates ($p < 0.01$) and 9 Spelling Retardates ($p < 0.05$). One of the "late"

control boys spoke clearly at 4 and the other at 5 years of age. Six Reading and 2 Spelling Retardates were 5 years old and 3 Reading and 2 Spelling Retardates were 6 years or older before speech was clear. Early articulatory defects were noted by the parents of both dyslexic groups significantly more frequently than by parents of the control groups, (Reading Retardates, $p < 0.001$, Spelling Retardates, $p < 0.02$). Difficulties in the use of language were noted more frequently by parents of the Reading Retardates ($p < 0.01$). While language difficulties were noted in a greater proportion of Spelling than of Reading Retardates, the comparison with Control 2 just failed to reach the 5 per cent level of significance. Although no answer to the questions on language difficulty other than "yes" or "no" was requested, many parents added comments about the nature of the difficulties. Such comments were almost entirely on grammatical structure including the incorrect formation of plural nouns and of tense and sometimes confusion in word order.

Table 22
Age at which Speech was Intelligible,
Early Articulatory Defects and Language
Difficulties noted by Parents

	Reading Retardates	Control 1	Spelling Retardates	Control 2
Age at which Speech was Intelligible				
less than 4 years	64·1%	97·6%	73·5%	96·3%
4 years or later	35·9%	2·4%***	26·5%	3·7%*
Mean age (years)	3·2	2·2	2·9	2·0
Number known	39	41	34	27
Number "Can't remember"	11	15	5	9
Number unknown	6	0	3	3
Articulatory Defects				
No	61·8%	94·6%	64·3%	90·0%
Yes	38·2%	5·4%***	35·7%	10·0%*
Number known	55	56	42	40
Language Difficulties				
No	78·2%	98·2%	71·4%	90·0%
Yes	21·8%	1·2%**	28·6%	10·0%
Number known	55	56	42	40
Chi-square 1 d.f.				

*Significant at the 5% level.
**Significant at the 1% level.
***Significant at the 0·1% level.

Articulation on Examination
Renfrew's Test of Articulation Attainment (see Chapter 5) was individually administered by a psychologist. The test was not given to 7 Reading Retardates and to 4 Spelling Retardates. Significant differences between the means of both dyslexic groups and their respective controls were found (Reading Retardates $p < 0.001$, Spelling Retardates $p < 0.05$). The extent of the difference between the Reading Retardates and Control 1 was not significantly greater than the difference between the Spelling Retardates and Control 2.

Using the criteria suggested by Miss Renfrew (included in the description of the test), articulation was defective in 17 Reading Retardates, 4 boys in Control 1, 8 Spelling Retardates and 3 boys in Control 2. In the control groups, the defect was classified as mild in all 7 cases, while the defect in 4 Reading and 2 Spelling Retardates was moderate or severe.

Table 23
Articulation Attainment Test

	Reading Retardates	Control 1	Spelling Retardates	Control 2
Mean score	96·8	98·8***	97·9	98·9*
SD	3·69	1·32	3·28	1·35

*Difference between means significant at the 5% level.
***Difference between means significant at the 0·1% level.

	Reading Retardates	Control 1	Spelling Retardates	Control 2
No articulatory defect	65·3%	92·9%	78·9%	92·9%
Poor or mildly defective articulation	26·5%	7·1%	15·8%	7·1%
Moderately or severely defective articulation	8·2%	0·0%	5·3%	0·0%
***Chi-square 1 d.f.	$p < 0.01$		$p > 0.05$	
Total number	49	56	38	42

The incidence of defective articulation in each control group is 7·1 per cent, which corresponds very closely with the incidence of 6·8 per cent observed in the Isle of Wight survey among the 147 control children aged 9 to 11 years (Rutter, Tizard and Whitmore, 1970). In the present study, the incidence of defective articulation among the dyslexic groups combined, 28·7 per cent, is considerably higher however than the 14 per cent observed by Rutter *et al.* among 86 children with specific reading difficulties.

Summary
Both dyslexic groups tend to be retarded in acquiring speech. The delay does not reach a significant level until sentences are used. Both dyslexic groups show a greater incidence of articulatory defects as noted by parents and on examination. Delayed speech and poor articulation are more marked among the Reading Retardates than among the Spelling Retardates, but the difference between them is not significant. Language difficulties were noted more frequently by the parents of both dyslexic groups but significantly so only in the case of the Reading Retardates.

Motor Development and Function
Information relating to motor development and motor function was obtained from two sources. The developmental history was provided by the parents on the Family Information Questionnaire and concerned the ages at which the boys sat up, crawled and walked unaided. Parents were asked also to record whether or not the boys had appeared to be clumsy. At the Centre, a

test of motor ability was administered by the psychologist. It was intended that Stott's revision of the Oseretsky test should be used but this could not be obtained until some months after the selection of children for this study had begun. A shortened form of the original Oseretsky already in use at the Centre, was employed until the Stott revision was received. Of the dyslexic children, 10 Reading Retardates and 10 Spelling Retardates were given this short form of the original Oseretsky Test of Motor Ability (see Chapter 5).

Motor Development

Many parents could not remember when their boys were first able to sit up but of the 42 who recorded "Can't remember," 16 added comments of "Average" or "Early." The majority of the boys in all groups for whom an age was given were sitting up at or before 8 months. No significant differences were found between Reading Retardates, Spelling Retardates and their respective control groups. Only 1 boy, a Reading Retardate, was unable to sit before he was 1 year old.

Table 24
Motor Development – Parental Report

	Reading Retardates	Control 1	Spelling Retardates	Control 2
Sitting Up				
less than 6 months	33·3%	22·7%	16·2%	19·2%
6 to 8 months	56·4%	61·4%	75·7%	69·2%
9 months or later	10·3%	15·9%	8·1%	11·5%
Chi-square 2 d.f.	$p > 0.05$		$p > 0.05$	
Number known	39	44	37	26
Number "Can't remember"	14	12	4	12
Number unknown	3	0	1	4
Walking Unaided				
less than 12 months	20·8%	11·1%	12·8%	13·5%
12 to 14 months	35·4%	61·1%	53·8%	48·6%
15 months or later	43·8%	27·8%	33·3%	37·8%
Chi-square 2 d.f.	$p < 0.05$		$p > 0.05$	
Number known	48	54	39	37
Number "Can't remember"	8	2	3	2
Number unknown	0	0	0	3
Clumsiness Noted				
No	76·8%	92·9%	71·4%	92·5%
Yes	23·2%	7·1%*	28·6%	7·5%*
Chi-square 1 d.f.	$p < 0.05$		$p > 0.05$	
Number known	56	56	42	40
Number unknown	0	0	0	2

Unfortunately parents were not asked whether their sons had or had not crawled but only the age at which they crawled. Whether any boys in this sample did not crawl remains unknown. An age was given for 34 Reading Retardates, 39 Control 1, 30 Spelling Retardates and 26 Control 2. No significant difference was found between either dyslexic group and its control. Few were not crawling by 12 months of age (5 Reading, 3 Spelling Retardates and 3 in each control group).

Only 15 parents could not remember when their boys began to walk independently and of these, eight added "average" and one added "late." The distributions of those walking unaided before 12 months, from 12 to 14 months and 15 months or later between the Reading Retardates and Control 1 differed significantly ($p < 0.05$) but not between the Spelling Retardates and Control 2. Almost 44 per cent of the Reading Retardates were not walking unaided until they were at least 15 months old.

All but the parents of two boys (Control 2) answered the question "Have you noticed any signs of clumsiness?" These had been noticed in 23·2 per cent of the Reading Retardates and 7·1 per cent of Control 1 ($p < 0.02$), in 28·6 per cent of the Spelling Retardates and 7·5 per cent of Control 2 ($p < 0.02$).

Motor Function on Examination

In five cases (namely, 2 Reading Retardates, 2 Spelling Retardates and 1 Control 1), a test was either not given or was incomplete. There are five subtests in the Stott Test of Motor Proficiency, Balance, Upper Limb Co-ordination, Whole Body Co-ordination, Manual Dexterity and Simultaneous Movement and three subtests in the shortened form of the Oseretsky Scale, Balance, Hand/Arm co-ordination (broadly comparable to Upper Limb Coordination) and Manual Dexterity. The number of children in each group whose performance was commensurate with chronological age in all subtests was calculated, and also an impairment score based on the criteria described in the manual. Since the shortened Oseretsky contains only three subtests the impairment scores for this were prorated to 5.

Performance on all subtests commensurate with chronological age was exhibited by 33·3 per cent of the Reading Retardates in contrast to 58·2 per cent of their Controls (the difference is significant at the 2 per cent level). Impairment scores of 4 or more are found more frequently among the Reading Retardates than among their controls. No significant differences are found between the Spelling Retardates and their controls.

Failure was more prevalent in some aspects of motor function than in others. More than a third of both Reading and Spelling Retardates, 35·2 per

Table 25
Test of Motor Proficiency

	Reading Retardates	Control 1	Spelling Retardates	Control 2
Performance commensurate with age on all subtests	33·3%	58·2%	50·0%	54·8%
Not commensurate	66·7%	41·8%*	50·0%	45·2%
Chi-square 1 d.f.	$p < 0.05$		$p > 0.05$	
Impairment score				
0 or 1	33·3%	69·1%***	50·0%	59·5%
2 or 3	38·9%	18·2%	25·0%	23·8%
4 and over	27·9%	12·7%	25·0%	16·7%
Chi-square 2 d.f.	$p < 0.001$		$p > 0.05$	
Total number	54	55	40	42

cent and 37·2 per cent respectively, failed on tasks of manual dexterity, in contrast to 16·4 per cent of Control 1 and 19·1 per cent of Control 2. The failure rate on tasks of balance was also higher in both dyslexic groups but more marked among the Reading Retardates (35·2 per cent Reading Retardates, 20 per cent Spelling Retardates, 12·7 per cent Control 1 and 7·1 per cent Control 2). Upper limb co-ordination tended to be poorer among the Reading Retardates (27·8 per cent as against 11 to 15 per cent in the other groups).

In the majority of Reading Retardates, performance was not entirely commensurate with chronological age, at all age levels but the number was significantly higher only at 8 and 9 years. A similar but not significant pattern was found among the younger Spelling Retardates. (Table 6, Appendix 1.)

Summary
No significant differences were found between dyslexics and controls with regard to the ages at which the boys were sitting up or crawling. Indeed the distribution of ages was very similar for each dyslexic group and its respective control group. However, in the case of the Reading Retardates there was a significantly greater number who were delayed in walking unaided. A significantly greater number of boys in both dyslexic groups had exhibited signs of clumsiness, according to their parents. On examination, only the Reading Retardates revealed a significantly greater number of boys whose performance on the motor test was below chronological age norms. Failure on the test tended to occur more frequently on tasks of manual dexterity and of balance It is possible that the Spelling Retardates had shown signs of some clumsiness at an early age but that co-ordination had improved by the time they were examined. It is also possible, of course, that the parental reports of clumsiness are unreliable, but if so the unreliability would appear to be greater in the case of the Spelling Retardates.

Finger Differentiation

The two tests of finger differentiation (described in Chapter 5) were administered and scored according to procedures adopted by Lady Clarke (personal communication) which differed slightly from those described by Kinsbourne and Warrington (1963 *a*). Lady Clarke had found that it was only at the lower percentile levels of 10 and 5 that retarded readers were distinguished from unselected children. The scores obtained by the boys in the present study were placed into one of three categories, those falling below the 5th percentile, those at the 10th or 5th percentile levels and those above the 10th percentile. Performance at these three levels is given for the dominant, that is the writing, and the non-dominant hands separately. It was possible that different results might be obtained for right-handers and left-handers, so these were separately computed. However, no differences were found and in the table below both right- and left-handers are combined.

On neither test of finger differentiation was a difference found between either dyslexic group and its control with respect to the dominant or to the non-dominant hands.

When performance on both tests was combined, 33 Reading Retardates, 39 of Control 1, 28 Spelling Retardates and 33 Control 2 responded at levels above the 10th percentile with both hands. Again no evidence is found of a greater incidence of finger agnosia among the dyslexic boys.

Table 26
Tests of Finger Differentiation

	Reading Retardates	Control 1	Spelling Retardates	Control 2
In-between Fingers Test				
Dominant hand				
Score above 10th percentile	77·8%	83·9%	79·5%	90·2%
Score at 10th or 5th percentile	9·3%	12·5%	10·3%	2·4%
Score below 5th percentile	13·0%	3·6%	10·3%	7·3%
Non-dominant hand				
Score above 10th percentile	81·5%	76·8%	84·6%	83·8%
Score at 10th or 5th percentile	5·5%	7·1%	5·1%	7·1%
Score below 5th percentile	13·0%	16·1%	10·3%	9·1%
Total number	54	56	39	41
One or Two Fingers Test				
Dominant hand				
Score above 10th percentile	88·7%	92·9%	94·1%	92·7%
Score at 10th or 5th percentile	3·8%	1·8%	2·9%	2·4%
Score below 5th percentile	7·5%	5·3%	2·9%	4·8%
Non-dominant hand				
Score above 10th percentile	88·7%	92·9%	100%	92·7%
Scores at 10th or 5th percentile	5·7%	3·5%	0%	2·4%
Score below 5th percentile	5·7%	3·5%	0%	4·8%
Total number	53	56	39	41

Chi-square 2 d.f. $p > 0.05$ in each comparison.

The number of boys whose performance was very poor is too small to draw any conclusion as to whether finger agnosia tended to occur more frequently at any particular age level. The abnormal responses were scattered fairly evenly over the entire age range in all groups.

Summary

There is no evidence, from either test of finger differentiation or from both tests considered together, to suggest that finger agnosia occurs with greater frequency among the dyslexic boys.

Right/Left Discrimination

Piaget (1928) described three stages in the evolution of concepts of right and left (see Chapter 2). The first two of these were examined, viz. the ability to identify the right and left of a child's own body and of a person facing him. Since the age range is 8 years to 12 years 11 months most children could be expected to identify right and left in relation to their own bodies.

A battery of 20 items was used (Swanson and Benton, 1955). The first ten require the subject to identify right and left parts of his own body with eyes open, the next six with his eyes closed and the last four questions require the child to identify right and left on the examiner who faces the subject. Analyses of variance were carried out on Total Scores, Own Body Eyes Open scores, Own Body Eyes Closed scores and Other Person scores.

Table 27
Test of Right/Left Discrimination

	Reading Retardates	Control 1	Spelling Retardates	Control 2
Mean total score	15·4	18·9***	17·7	18·3
Mean score Own body eyes open	7·9	9·6***	9·2	9·4
Mean score Own body eyes closed	5·0	5·9***	5·6	5·8
Mean score Other person	2·5	3·5***	2·9	3·1
Total number	52	56	40	42

***Difference between means significant at the 0·1% level.

Highly significant differences were found between Reading Retardates and Control 1, on Own Body Eyes Open ($p < 0.001$), Own Body Eyes Closed ($p < 0.001$), Other Person ($p < 0.001$) and Total Scores ($p < 0.001$). None of the comparisons for Spelling Retardates and Control 2 reached a level of significance.

The differences between Reading Retardates and Control 1 were significantly greater than the differences between Spelling Retardates and Control 2 with regard to Own Body Eyes Open ($p < 0.05$) and Total Scores ($p < 0.01$) only. On the more difficult tasks, Own Body Eyes Closed and Other Person, the differences were not significant.

Thus, while right/left confusion is marked among the Reading Retardates only, it is only the simpler level of right/left discrimination and total scores which significantly distinguish them from the Spelling Retardates.

It was possible that difficulties might be more apparent among the younger boys than among the older ones. Inspection of the means obtained at 8, 9, 10, 11 and 12 years (see Table 7, Appendix 1) suggests that at all three levels of right/left discrimination the Reading Retardates were not reaching near perfect scores until 12 years of age whereas the boys in Control 1 obtained near perfect scores from the age of 8 years. Among the Spelling Retardates, near perfect scores were common from the age of 9 years on Own Body items but not until 10 years of age on Other Person items. In Control 2, the Other Person mean at 8 years is as low as that of the Reading Retardates. Three boys in this control group made no score on this part of the test. One was retarded by 12 months in Spelling (IQ 115) one by 6 months in spelling (IQ 115) and the third was reading and spelling at chronological age level (IQ 133).

Swanson and Benton give the mean total score for unselected 8-year-olds as 17·3, standard deviation 1·99, and for unselected 9-year-olds as 18·0, standard deviation 1·82. The numbers of boys obtaining 15 points or less at 8 years, 16 points or less at 9 years, 17 points or less at 10 years and 18 points or less at 11 and 12 years, were calculated. At each of these age levels a significantly greater number of Reading Retardates than boys in Control 1 obtained low scores. No significant differences were found between Spelling Retardates and their control group except at 11 or 12 years, when perfect scores were obtained by all 7 Spelling Retardates but by only 3 of their control group.

Right/left confusion was found throughout the age range of 8 years to 12 years 11 months among the Reading Retardates. The only age at which nearly half of the Spelling Retardates revealed directional confusions was at 8 years and this was not significant.

Table 28
Right/Left Discrimination: Total Score in Relation to Chronological Age

		Reading Retardates	Control 1	Spelling Retardates	Control 2
8 years	15 or less	5	0	5	3
	16 or more	4	8	6	9
				$p > 0.05$	
9 years	16 or less	10	2	1	1
	17 or more	0	10	7	11
		$p < 0.01$		$p > 0.05$	
10 years	17 or less	6	4	4	4
	18 or more	9	13	7	9
		$p < 0.05$		$p > 0.05$	
11 and	18 or less	9	1	0	3
12 years	19 or 20	9	18	7	3
		$p < 0.01$		$p < 0.05$	

Summary
On the test of right/left discrimination, significant differences were found between the Reading Retardates and Control 1 on each part of the test and on total scores. No differences were found between the Spelling Retardates and their controls. Only the simplest level of right/left differentiation and total scores significantly distinguish Reading from Spelling Retardates. Confusion is significantly frequent at all age levels among the Reading Retardates. There appears to be some tendency for confusion to be more prevalent among the youngest Spelling Retardates but the numbers are small and do not reach a level of significance.

Auditory Discrimination

Wepman's Test of Auditory Discrimination was given (see Chapter 5). The ability to discriminate speech sounds increases with age (Templin, 1957). According to Wepman (1958), 4 or more errors on this test indicate some degree of difficulty in children of 8 years +. Four errors could be made by confusing "v" and "th" and "f" and "th" only, and these were found to occur so frequently among dyslexics and controls, that a score of 5 or more is regarded here as indicative of a difficulty. Dyslexics scoring 5 or more had been referred for audiometry and included only when the audiogram was normal.

There is no significant difference between the mean scores of either of the dyslexic groups and their respective controls, nor is there any difference between Reading and Spelling Retardates. Also calculated were the numbers of boys making 0—4 errors and 5 or more errors. An almost identical distribution is found among Reading Retardates and Control 1. Although twice as many Retardates as their controls obtained scores outside the normal limit, the numbers are small and the difference not significant.

An examination was made of the distribution of the sounds which were confused. Confusions between "v" and "th," "f" and "th" occurred commonly in all groups. Likewise errors in distinguishing between "m" and "n," "k" and "p" were found in all groups but with considerably less frequency. All sounds confused by boys in the control groups were also confused by the dyslexic boys, but some pairs of sounds seemed to cause difficulty either only or almost entirely to the dyslexics. These included the short vowels a—e; e—i; and the consonants b—d; d—g; th—sh; sh—th.

Table 29
Test of Auditory Discrimination

	Reading Retardates	Control 1	Spelling Retardates	Control 2
Score				
0—4	82.1%	80.4%	70.7%	85.7%
5 +	17.9%	19.6%	29.3%	14.3%
Mean score	3.4	3.0	3.3	2.9
Total number	56	56	41	42

No statistically significant differences.

Summary
No differences were found between either dyslexic group and its control group in the mean number of errors made nor in the numbers of boys whose scores fell outside normal limits. However, some pairs of sounds caused difficulty only or largely to the dyslexics.

Sound Blending
The test comprised 20 familiar words, 5 each of two, three, four and five letters. Each word was sounded very slowly, enunciated letter by letter. After listening and repeating these, the child had to say what the word was. Scores range from 1 to 5. The task is complex involving the perception of the sounds, their accurate reproduction, the ability to hold the sequence in correct order and to blend the sounds into whole words. In attempting to read an unknown word, a child relies on his ability to decode symbols into sounds, to remember these in sequence and to synthesize them.

The inability to blend sounds could be regarded as a consequence of poor reading or alternatively, as Leroy-Bussion and Dupessy's (1969) work might suggest, the poor reading may result, to some extent at least, from a difficulty in blending.

Among the Reading Retardates difficulties in blending sounds were very common. Approximately 2 out of 3 could not reliably blend more than three to four sounds compared with fewer than one-quarter of their controls ($p < 0.001$). The difference between the mean scores for these groups was also highly significant ($p < 0.001$).

The Spelling Retardates, who were not so severely retarded in reading, also differed from their control group with regard to mean scores but at a very much lower level of significance ($p < 0.05$). Fewer Spelling Retardates than their controls were able to blend more than four sounds reliably but the difference was not significant. No difference was found between Reading and Spelling Retardates.

Specific Dyslexia

Table 30
Test of Sound Blending

	Reading Retardates	Control 1	Spelling Retardates	Control 2
Score				
1 to 3·8	65·5%	23·2%	56·1%	38·1%
4 to 5	34·5%	76·8%	43·9%	61·9%
Chi-square 1 d.f	$p < 0·01$		$p > 0·05$	
Mean score	3·5	4·3***	3·8	4·2*
Total number	55	56	41	42

*Difference between means significant at the 5% level.
***Difference between means significant at the 0·1% level.

Table 31
Improvement in Sound Blending with Increasing Age

		Dyslexics	Controls
8 years	less than 4	81·0%	40·0%
	4 or more	19·0%	60·0%
9 years	less than 4	75·0%	37·5%
	4 or more	25·0%	62·5%
10 years	less than 4	62·0%	35·0%
	4 or more	38·0%	65·0%
11 and	less than 4	34·6%	18·5%
12 years	4 or more	65·4%	81·5%
Total number		96	98

The ability to blend an increasing number of sounds increases with age, even among the controls whose reading standards were high. In Table 31 both dyslexic and both control groups are combined. At each age level are shown the numbers of boys scoring less than 4, in practice reliably blending three to four sounds, and those scoring 4 to 5 and blending four to five sounds. By the age of 11 or 12 years, the majority of the dyslexics blend four to five sounds but a majority of the controls can do so at 8 years. Among dyslexics and controls, the percentage of boys scoring 4 or more increases from the age of 8 years upwards with a sharper increase after the age of 10 years.

Summary
The mean scores on a test of blending sounds are significantly lower in the case of both Reading and Spelling Retardates but at different levels of significance (Reading Retardates $p < 0·001$, Spelling Retardates $p < 0·05$). Approximately two-thirds of the Reading Retardates could not reliably blend more than three to four sounds.

The number of boys able to blend four to five sounds increases with increasing age in both dyslexics and controls. But whereas it is not until the age of 11 years that a majority of dyslexic boys show this ability, among the controls a majority can do so from the age of 8 years upwards.

Visual Retention

The ability to remember and reproduce a complex visual pattern is involved in spelling, especially those words which are phonically irregular.

Visual retention was examined by giving Benton's Test of Visual Retention, Form C, Administration A, in accordance with the instructions in the manual. Norms are provided taking into account both chronological age and IQ for the number of correctly reproduced designs and for the number of errors.

Table 32 gives the means and standard deviations for the number of correctly reproduced designs and the number of errors made. The mean

Table 32
Benton's Visual Retention Test

	Reading Retardates	Control 1	Spelling Retardates	Control 2
Designs Correct				
Mean number	5·6	6·6**	6·1	7·0
SD	2·03	1·85	1·64	4·35
Errors				
Mean number	6·5	4·9**	6·3	5·8
SD	3·20	3·86	4·00	4·09
Designs Correct	No.	No.	No.	No.
At or above expected score	44	35	30	33
Below expected score	12	21	12	9
Errors				
At or below expected score	45	46	30	31
Above expected score	11	10	12	11
Total number of boys	56	56	42	42

**Difference between means significant at the 1% level.

number of correct designs is lower and the mean number of errors higher for the Reading and Spelling Retardates than for their respective controls. The differences between Reading Retardates and Control 1 are significant at the 1 per cent level but not significant between Spelling Retardates and Control 2. No significant difference was found between the Reading and Spelling Retardates.

Comparisons based on the number of boys whose scores were at or above the "expected" level and those whose scores were below the "expected" level are not significant however. In Control 1, 21 boys failed to reach the norm on designs correct but only 9 of these also failed to reach the norm on errors. Of the 12 Reading Retardates failing on designs, 9 failed on errors also. Of the 15 boys in the control groups whose performance was below expectation on both designs correct and errors, 10 achieved a spelling age below chronological age, the spelling quotient of 7 being less than 80.

The use of the Full Scale IQ in determining whether performance is at or below the norms provided poses certain problems when some subtests present specific difficulties and lower the IQ even a little. A somewhat different result might have been obtained had, for example, a shortened form of the WISC been used.

Summary
On Benton's Visual Retention Test, the Reading Retardates produced fewer designs correctly ($p < 0.01$) and made a greater number of errors than their

control group ($p < 0.01$). No differences were found with regard to the
Spelling Retardates. When both chronological age and IQ were taken into
account, there were no differences in the numbers falling at or below the
"expected" level in any comparison.

Laterality

The tests of hand dominance, eye and foot preference are described in
Chapter 5. Cross-laterality and hand-eye-foot correspondence were derived
from the results of these. It was possible that children examined at the
Centre might include a spuriously high number with atypical laterality
patterns and that this would be reflected in the frequencies found in the
dyslexic groups. Each dyslexic and control group was therefore compared
with all boys examined at the Centre while this sample was being collected.
The dyslexic boys who are the subjects of this investigation are excluded from
"other Centre" cases. In three of these comparisons significant differences
were found. The Reading Retardates differed from other Centre cases in the
distribution of strong right-handedness, strong left-handedness and ambilaterality, there being among the Reading Retardates a greater proportion of
ambilaterals and fewer strongly right-handed boys ($p < 0.02$). The Spelling
Retardates included a greater proportion of cross-lateral boys ($p < 0.01$) and
a greater proportion in whom hand, eye and foot were not concordant
($p < 0.01$) than other Centre cases. None of the differences between either
control group and other Centre cases was significant.

A significantly greater number of Reading Retardates than boys in Control
1 wrote with the left hand ($p < 0.05$) but no difference was found between
Spelling Retardates and Control 2.

The test of simultaneous writing was scored in terms of strong right,
moderate right, ambilateral, moderate left and strong left. The intermediate
categories have been combined and described as "Ambilateral." The Reading
Retardates included fewer more strongly right-handed and more ambilaterals
than their control group ($p < 0.05$) and while the number of strongly left-
handed boys is greater, it is not markedly so. The Reading Retardates differ
from their controls and also from other Centre boys.

The consistent use of one eye on both tests of eye-preference was recorded as either "right" or "left" as the case may be. All other responses were
recorded as "mixed." In keeping with many previous investigations (Clark,
1957; Harris, 1957; Pringle, Butler and Davie, 1966), left-eyedness was found
in approximately one-third of each group, dyslexic and control, and other
Centre boys. In this study, it is the incidence of right- and mixed-eyedness
which varies. The distribution of right-, left- and mixed-eyedness reaches a
significant level only with regard to the Spelling Retardates and their controls
($p < 0.05$).

Two tests of foot preference are used, kicking and hopping. Performance
was scored "right," "left" or "mixed" as for eye-dominance. The number of
consistently left-footed boys in all groups was small. Indeed none was found
in Control 2. In the comparisons reported, right and left are combined. The
distribution of definite and indeterminate foot dominance was similar in all
groups with the exception of Control 1. Nevertheless the difference between
the Reading Retardates and Control 1 falls short of the 5 per cent level of
significance. No difference was found between Spelling Retardates and Control 2

Table 33
Hand, Eye and Foot Preferences

	Reading Retardates	Control 1	Spelling Retardates	Control 2	Centre
Handedness					
writing – right	73%	91%*	79%	90%	82%
writing – left	27%	9%	21%	10%	18%
Number	55	56	42	42	163
Chi-square 1 d.f.	$p < 0.05$		$p > 0.05$		
Strongly right-handed	50%	75%*	59%	81%	66%[1]
Strongly left-handed	9%	5%	12%	5%	14%
Ambilateral	41%	20%	29%	14%	20%
Number	54	56	41	42	146
Chi-square 2 d.f.	$p < 0.05$		$p > 0.05$		
Eyedness					
right	53%	57%	39%	62%*	43%
left	33%	30%	37%	31%	39%
mixed	15%	13%	24%	7%	18%
Number	55	56	41	42	164
Chi-square 2 d.f.	$p < 0.05$		$p > 0.05$		
Footedness					
right	47% ⎫	70% ⎫	45% ⎫	55% ⎫	46% ⎫
left	7% ⎭	4% ⎭	8% ⎭	0% ⎭	14% ⎭
mixed	45%	27%	48%	45%	40%
Number	55	56	40	42	164
Chi-square 1 d.f.	$p < 0.05$		$p > 0.05$		
Cross-laterality					
Not cross-lateral	50%	59%	32%	62%*	54%[2]
Cross-lateral	50%	41%	68%	38%	46%
Number	54	56	41	42	162
Chi-square 1 d.f.	$p < 0.05$		$p > 0.05$		
Hand, eye and foot					
Unilaterally concordant	31%	45%	12%	43%**	33%[3]
Not concordant	69%	55%	88%	57%	67%
Number	55	56	41	42	164
Chi-square 1 d.f.	$p < 0.01$		$p > 0.05$		

Percentages to the nearest whole number.
[1] Centre v Reading Retardates chi-square 2 d.f. $p < 0.02$.
[2] Centre v Spelling Retardates chi-square 1 d.f. $p < 0.01$.
[3] Centre v Spelling Retardates chi-square 1 d.f. $p < 0.01$.

Cross-laterality is the term used to describe a lack of correspondence between the dominant hand and eye such as right-handedness with left-eyedness. Boys who wrote with the right hand and used the right eye consistently on both tests of eye-dominance and those who wrote with the left hand and used the left eye consistently, were recorded as "not cross-lateral," all others are described as "cross-lateral." On these criteria, the incidence of cross-laterality is high in all groups including all Centre boys. Of the Spelling Retardates 67 per cent were cross-lateral in contrast to 38 per cent of the boys in control 2 ($p < 0.02$). They also differed significantly from other Centre boys. There is no significant difference between Reading Retardates and their controls.

Concordant dominance of hand, eye and foot is a feature not commonly investigated. Complete concordance on either the right or left side was found in less than 50 per cent of all groups, dyslexic and control, and other Centre cases. There was only 1 subject with complete left-sided dominance (Reading Retardate). The Spelling Retardates include a significantly greater number of boys with incomplete dominance than either other Centre boys ($p < 0.01$) or their control group ($p < 0.01$). Indeed in only 5 Spelling Retardates, 12 per cent, was dominance completely unilaterally concordant.

Summary

The incidence of left-handedness, of left-eyedness, of left-footedness, of cross-laterality and of mixed hand-eye-foot dominance tended to be higher among Centre cases (excluding the Reading and Spelling Retardates) than that found in the control groups but in no instance was a significant difference found. The Reading Retardates included a greater number of left-handed writers than their control group ($p < 0.05$), fewer strongly right-handed boys and more ambilaterals than both their control group ($p < 0.05$) and other Centre boys ($p < 0.02$). The Spelling Retardates included fewer right-eyed boys and a greater number of mixed eye-dominance that their controls ($p < 0.05$). Cross-laterality was found more frequently among the Spelling Retardates than their control group ($p < 0.05$) and other Centre boys ($p < 0.01$). In only 12 per cent of the Spelling Retardates was hand-eye-foot dominance concordant compared with 43 per cent of their controls ($p < 0.01$) and 33 per cent ($p < 0.01$) of other Centre boys.

8

Neurological Examination and Medical History

By Alfred White Franklin

Neurological Examination

A routine examination of the central nervous system was carried out on classical lines on all children examined at the Centre. No gross deviations from normal were expected and had such been found the child would have been excluded from the group. With regard to the refined examination of motor function, co-ordination and ability to carry out correctly simultaneous movements of different limbs, these were left to the psychologist and are described in Chapter 5. Two methods of examination revealed during the years of the study abnormalities of significance. These were firstly getting the supine patient to stroke the heel along the opposite shin from knee to ankle (knee to ankle test) and secondly watching the pupils as the patient's eyes followed the examiner's finger held about one foot in front of him and moved horizontally to right and to left (nystagmoid movement).

Most children examined were able to produce a smooth knee to ankle test, but a few moved the heel jerkily down the opposite shin and were unable to control the movement. The jerky movement was found on both sides and its presence is recorded as a positive test. This manœuvre is included in the classical examination of the central nervous system as a test for inco-ordination and/or ataxia. Its proper performance depends on the integrity of both sensory and motor pathways and of a normal organization of and connection between the impulses received and those sent out. Gross cerebellar disease, loss of position sense, of body image as well as motor weakness could produce an abnormal test result. Such gross lesions were not present in the children studied. Not all of them showed evidence of inco-ordination on the Stott-Oseretsky tests. No explanation is offered for this abnormal finding.

Most children too had good control of eye movements when following the moving finger whether the finger was moved slowly or quickly. A test was recorded as negative when the eyeballs moved to a complete halt. In a positive test there was a short series of nystagmoid movements at the extremity of the lateral deviation, never persistent, sometimes only in one direction and sometimes in both. No extra movements occurred when the examiner's finger stopped level with the child's nose. The neurological basis for the nystagmoid movements is unknown, but Dr Hood (personal communication, 1970)

75

reports a similar finding in dyslexic children, which he has demonstrated on electro-oculograms. A positive knee to ankle test and the nystagmoid eye movements have been shown to be of significance in the study. The absence of explanation as to the neurological basis for the abnormal results is deplored. Further study might shed light on the neurological basis for the dyslexia.

Tendon Reflexes. No significant difference was found between the groups of those with normal and those with abnormal tendon reflexes (diminished, increased, exaggerated, with reinforcement). An exaggerated response and response with reinforcement occurred only in 3 dyslexic boys (2 Reading, 1 Spelling Retardate).

Knee to Ankle Test. The incidence of a positive knee to ankle test was higher among both dyslexic groups, but the difference was significant only between Spelling Retardates and Control ($p < 0.02$).

Nystagmoid Eye Movements. There was a higher incidence of nystagmoid movements in both dyslexic groups, significant only between Spelling Retardates and Controls ($p < 0.001$) and more marked on deviation to the left ($p < 0.001$) than to the right ($p < 0.01$). It was found on deviation to the right only in 2 boys (1 Spelling Retardate and 1 Control 2) and to the left only in 12 boys (2 Reading Retardates, 5 Spelling Retardates, 3 Control 1 and 2 Control 2). On deviation of the eyes to both right and left it occurred more frequently among the dyslexic boys (6 Reading and 8 Spelling Retardates) than among the Controls (3 Control 1 and 1 Control 2). No reason is suggested for the presence of these movements nor for their higher frequency on deviation of the eyes to the left.

Table 34
Tendon Reflexes and the Knee to Ankle Test

	Reading Retardates		Control 1		Spelling Retardates		Control 2	
Tendon Reflexes								
Normal	43	81·1%	46	85·2%	34	82·9%	38	90·5%
Diminished	1		1		1		1	
Increased	7	18·9%	7	14·8%	5	17·1%	3	9·5%
Exaggerated	2		0		0		0	
With reinforcement	0		0		1		0	
Number recorded	53		54		41		42	
Knee to Ankle Test								
Negative	33	73·3%	47	88·7%	20	71·4%	40	95·2%*
Positive	12	26·7%	6	11·3%	8	28·6%	2	4·8%
Number recorded	45		53		28		42	

*Chi-square 1 d.f. significant at the 5% level.

Table 35
Nystagmoid Eye Movements

Nystagmoid movement on deviation to	Reading Retardates	Control 1	Spelling Retardates	Control 2
Right and Left				
Absent	78·9%	88·7%	53·3%	90·5%***
Present	21·1%	11·3%	46·7%	9·5%
Right only				
Absent	84·2%	94·3%	69·0%	95·2%**
Present	15·8%	5·7%	31·0%	4·8%
Left only				
Absent	78·9%	88·7%	56·7%	92·9%***
Present	21·1%	11·3%	43·3%	7·1%
Number recorded	38	53	30	42

**Chi-square 1 d.f. significant at the 1% level.
***Chi-square 1 d.f. significant at the 0·1% level.

Illnesses

In completing the Family Questionnaire, parents were asked to state whether specified illnesses had occurred before the age of 5 years (pre-school), after the age of 5 (school age) and, if age could not be remembered, to state "yes" or "no."

The illnesses included common childhood infections such as chicken-pox, mumps, measles, all often contracted during the early school years. Dyslexic boys were excluded when they had had protracted periods of absence during the first two years of schooling, a factor which may contribute to the slightly higher incidence of many complaints over 5 years of age among the control groups.

None was epileptic. Two boys (Control 1) had had poliomyelitis during the pre-school years. One (Control 1) had had encephalitis over 5 years of age. One Reading Retardate had Rheumatic Fever over 5 years of age. Convulsions and fits had been experienced by 3 boys before going to school (1 Reading, 1 Spelling Retardate, 1 Control 1). Three boys (1 Reading, 2 Spelling Retardates) had had spells of fainting over 5 years of age. Eight boys had jaundice (apart from neonatal jaundice), all during the pre-school years (4 Reading, 3 Spelling Retardates, 1 Control 1).

No significant difference was found between those who had had, or had not had, chicken-pox, mumps, measles or german measles.(Table 8, Appendix 1.)

Accidents

As clumsiness, or poor motor co-ordination, is reported to be more frequent among children with a specific reading disability (Rutter, Tizard and Whitmore, 1970) a greater accident proneness and an increased incidence of accidents might be expected among them. The percentage of Reading Retardates with a history of an accident of any kind under 5 years is identical with that of Control 1, but accidents were reported in three times as many Control 2 boys as Spelling Retardates.

The proportion of boys having accidents after 5 years of age in Control 2 is also slightly higher. None of the differences is significant. (Table 9, Appendix 1.)

Bones had been broken most commonly over the age of 5 (20 boys, 7 Reading, 1 Spelling Retardate, 8 Control 1, 4 Control 2), while injuries involving the head were most common under 5 years (22 boys, 7 Reading, 1 Spelling Retardate, 7 Control 1, 9 Control 2). The injuries were mainly minor cuts and bruises. Only 1 child (Control 1) had been burned severely under 5 years. These accidents do not appear to have played any real part in producing dyslexia.

Asthma

Ten boys had, or had had, asthma (4 Reading, 2 Spelling Retardates, 4 Control 1), which had developed during school years in 4 (2 Reading, 1 Spelling Retardates, 1 Control 1). The incidence of asthma in the whole group (5·1 per cent) is slightly higher than the 3·6 per cent reported in boys by Pringle, Butler and Davie (1966). It was slightly more common among dyslexic boys than among controls, but not significantly so. This must not be interpreted as excluding asthma from being the possible result of school strain leading to school absence in any individual boy. (Table 10, Appendix 1.)

Eczema

Eczema was reported in 26 boys. In 3, age was not specified but 15 of the remaining 23 suffered from eczema before the age of 3 years (4 Reading Retardates, 4 Control 1, 4 Spelling Retardates and 3 Control 2). In 18 boys eczema was a recurring ailment but again there was no significant difference between the groups (5 Reading Retardates, 5 Control 1, 4 Spelling Retardates, 4 Control 2).(Table 10, Appendix 1.)

Headaches

Parents reported that 43 boys had at some time complained of headaches, 12 between the ages of 3 to 5 years (5 Reading Retardates, 1 Control 1, 3 Spelling Retardates, 3 Control 2), and 21 from 6 to 12 years (7 Reading Retardates, 1 Control 1, 4 Spelling Retardates, 9 Control 2). The age was not specified for 10 boys.

Although a greater number of Reading Retardates than of Control 1 had complained of headaches, the highest frequency was found in Control 2, surprisingly since the stress arising from a learning disability might be expected to cause headaches more frequently among the dyslexics, if it be correct to blame headaches on strain.(Table 10, Appendix 1.)

Bed-wetting

Bed-wetting after 5 years of age was found to occur in 12·1 per cent of 4,059 7-year-old boys in the population studied by Pringle, Butler and Davie (1966). 75 per cent of the Reading Retardates and 75·5 per cent of their Controls were dry at night by the age of 3 years, as were 67·5 per cent of Spelling Retardates and 76·8 per cent of their Controls. The differences between the groups of those dry by 3 years and those dry later are not significant. A further 8·9 per cent Reading Retardates, 18·8 per cent Control 1, 17·5 per cent Spelling Retardates and 12·8 per cent Control 2 were dry at night by the age of 5 years. Bed-wetting after the age of 5 years occurred in 16 per cent Reading Retardates, 5·7 per cent Control 1, 15 per cent Spelling Retardates and 10·3 per cent Control 2. Compared with the boys in Pringle, Butler and Davie's survey the incidence is lower among both control groups and higher among the dyslexics. Many parents of dyslexic boys reported that bed-wetting tended to recur during term time rather than during holidays.

Soiling

The National Survey quoted above (Pringle, Butler and Davie, 1966) indicated that 1·8 per cent of 4,059 boys had not achieved bowel control by the age of 4 years. In the Isle of Wight Survey (Rutter, Tizard and Whitmore, 1970) the prevalence of soiling among boys aged 10 to 12 years was slightly less, 1·3 per cent. In this study, 7 out of the 192 boys, about whom information was given, were still soiling occasionally after 5 years of age, i.e. 3·6 per cent, which is higher than the incidence found in the national survey. Two were still occasionally encopretic between 9 to 11 years (1 Reading Retardate, 1 Control 2). No significant difference was found between dyslexics and controls.

Table 36
Bed-wetting and Soiling

	Reading Retardates	Control 1	Spelling Retardates	Control 2
Bed-wetting				
Dry at night by 3 years	75·0%	75·5%	67·5%	76·9%
Not dry till 3 to 5 years	8·9%	18·8%	17·5%	12·8%
Not dry till 6 to 8 years	8·9%	3·8%	7·5%	7·7%
Not dry till 9 to 11 years	7·1%	1·9%	7·5%	2·6%
Total number	56	53	40	39
Soiling				
No soiling after 3 years	92·7%	87·3%	95·0%	97·5%
No soiling after 3 to 5 years	1·8%	7·3%	5·0%	0·0%
No soiling after 6 to 8 years	3·6%	5·4%	0·0%	0·0%
Still occasionally soiling, 9 to 11 years	1·8%	0·0%	0·0%	2·5%
Total number	55	55	40	40

Chi-square 1 d.f. $p > 0.05$

Emotional strain, whether at home in the family, or at school in the educational setting, is usually regarded as important in the aetiology of asthma and eczema, as well as in the acquisition of sphincter control. In identifying the part played by dyslexia, great care is needed. Family disappointment over school failure can be strongly felt and strongly expressed. Family strain, of whatever nature, is known to interfere with educational progress. Whatever is proved or not proved by statistical studies with their correct controls, the doctor, the psychologist, the teacher and the parent would be indeed unwise not to explore all these interactions in any child with serious educational problems.

Perinatal Factors

Information about perinatal conditions was obtained from the parents (*see* Family Information Questionnaire, Appendix 2) and an obstetric report from hospitals was also available in 111 cases. The mother's description of a normal home birth was accepted, and birth was assumed to be normal on the mother's report when no report could be obtained from the hospital or nursing home.

Place of birth. Hospital confinements were commonest in all groups, with relatively few babies, between 5 to 14 per cent in each group, born in nursing homes. Between 69 and 83 per cent of boys in each of the four groups were born in hospital or nursing home and there were no significant differences between either dyslexic group and its control with regard to the numbers born at home or in hospital or nursing home. (Table 11, Appendix 1.)

Single or multiple birth. Information was given about 194 boys of whom 190 were single born. The remaining 4 were twins (1 Reading Retardate, 3 Spelling Retardates) 3 of the 4 being born second. Twin births occur in about 1 in 80 pregnancies and although the number of Spelling Retardates is very small, an incidence of 3 twins out of 41 boys is higher than might be expected.

Birth weight. The mean birth weight for each group, and also the number of boys whose birth weights were 5 lb 8 oz or less, over 5 lb 8 oz to 7 lb 8 oz, or over 7 lb 8 oz are given in Table 37. Six boys, including 2 of the 4 twins, were premature by weight, that is, 5 lb 8 oz or less at birth. All of

Table 37
Birth Weight, Single and Multiple Births

	Reading Retardates	Control 1	Spelling Retardates	Control 2
Mean birth weight (oz)	125·6	120·2	120·7	121·9
Less than 5lb 8oz	2	0	4	0
5lb 9oz to 7lb 8oz	20	31	17	21
7lb 9oz and over	33	25	21	19
Total number	55	56	42	40
Single birth	55	56	38	39
Multiple birth	1	0	3	0
Total number	56	56	41	39

No statistically significant differences.

them were among the dyslexics (2 Reading, 4 Spelling Retardates). Boys of
birth weight over 7 lb 8 oz were more numerous among the dyslexics
particularly the Reading Retardates, fewer of whom were first-born. First-born
infants tend to weigh less at birth than subsequently-born infants.

Differences between mean birth weights were not significant.

Maternal Reports of Pregnancy and Delivery

Mothers were asked in the Family Information Questionnaire to record
whether they had had any illnesses during pregnancy and, if so, to state what
these were. In ten cases this information was not given (5 Reading, 2 Spelling
Retardates and 3 Control 2). Altogether 37 mothers reported that they had
had some illness, these including pernicious vomiting, toxaemia, hypertension,
oedema, diabetes mellitus, haemorrhage, thrombosis, pneumonia, pleurisy,
asthma, bronchitis, Asian 'flu, chicken-pox, rubella, mumps, cystitis, colitis.
Of the 37, 17 were mothers of Reading Retardates, 6 of Control 1 ($p < 0.01$),
10 of Spelling Retardates and 4 of Control 2 ($p > 0.05$).

There were significantly greater numbers of mothers with complaints of
pregnancy illnesses when the whole group of dyslexics was compared with the
controls ($p < 0.01$) and when reading retardates were compared with their
controls ($p < 0.01$). The fact that the illnesses involved included chronic
medical conditions like asthma and diabetes mellitus as well as toxaemia of
pregnancy makes it unlikely that there was any physical effect on the
developing foetus. Possibly the mothers of dyslexics who were worried
enough to seek help for their children were more accurate in their recording
than the mothers of controls.

Table 38
Maternal Reports of Pregnancy and Delivery

	Reading Retardates	Control 1	Spelling Retardates	Control 2
Pregnancy				
No illness reported	34	50**	30	35
Some illness reported	17	6	10	4
Total number	51	56	40	39
Delivery				
Normal	40	44	31	25
Otherwise †	13	11	8	13
Total number	53	55	39	38

**Chi-square 1 d.f. significant at 1% level.
†Otherwise includes caesarian, breech, P.O.P., forceps and other.

Delivery. Mothers were asked to record whether delivery was normal,
caesarian, breech, P.O.P. or other and whether forceps had been used. This
information was not given by eleven Mothers (3 Reading, 3 Spelling Retardates, 1 Control 1 and 4 Control 2). Delivery was stated by 45 Mothers to be
other than normal (13 Reading Retardates, 11 Control 1, 8 Spelling Retardates, 13 Control 2). These differences were not significant. One point of
interest that emerged was the disparity between the mother's report and that
of the hospital. When the hospital had grounds for anxiety this was always

Specific Dyslexia

conveyed to the mother, but a number of mothers regarded their confinements as abnormal when there was no medical or obstetrical reason for their doing so.

Table 39
Concordance between Hospital and Maternal Reports of Perinatal History: Dyslexics and Controls Combined

| | Maternal Report | | |
	Normal	*Abnormal*	*Total*
Hospital Report			
Normal	46	34	80
Abnormal	4	20	24
Total number	50	54	104

Neonatal period. Details of the presence of specific illnesses, feeding difficulties and persistent crying occurring during the first four weeks of life were requested from the parents. Convulsions or Fits were not reported for any child, dyslexic or control.

Jaundice. Twelve boys were reported to have had jaundice (5 Reading, 3 Spelling Retardates, 3 Control 1 and 1 Control 2). Although jaundice occurred twice as frequently among the dyslexics combined, this distribution is not significant ($p > 0.05$).

High temperatures. These had been recorded in only 3 dyslexics (1 Reading, 2 Spelling Retardates).

Feeding difficulties. These were reported in 24 boys (5 Reading, 2 Spelling Retardates, 8 Control 1 and 9 Control 2). Feeding difficulties were reported more frequently in the control groups but the distribution is not significant ($p > 0.05$).

Persistent crying. Twenty-one boys were said to have cried persistently during the first 4 weeks (8 Reading, 3 Spelling Retardates, 7 Control 1 and 3 Control 2). The distribution is very similar between each dyslexic group and its control group ($p > 0.05$).

Table 40
Hospital Report on Rh Factor and Jaundice at Birth: 83 Boys

	Reading Retardates	*Control 1*	*Spelling Retardates*	*Control 2*
Mother Rh−				
Yes	21·7%	4·2%	17·6%	0%
No	78·3%	95·8%	82·4%	100%
Total number	23	24	17	19
Baby Jaundiced				
Yes	4·7%	0%	13·3%	5·3%
No	95·3%	100%	86·7%	94·7%
Total number	21	24	15	19

No statistically significant differences.

Hospital obstetric reports. Of the 111 hospital reports obtained, 83 specifically stated whether or not mother's blood contained an Rh negative factor. Mother's blood was Rh– in 9 cases (5 Reading Retardates, 1 Control 1 and 3 Spelling Retardates).

Only 4 babies were jaundiced and in only 1 was jaundice also reported by mother (Spelling Retardate). Of the 4 who had jaundice, 3 were dyslexics (1 Reading, 2 Spelling Retardates and 1 Control 2).

Perinatal conditions were judged abnormal in 25 boys (6 Reading Retardates, 8 Control 1, 7 Spelling Retardates, 4 Control 2). The distribution of abnormal and normal between each dyslexic group and its control is in both comparisons not significant.

Table 41

Physician's Assessment of Perinatal Conditions

	Reading Retardates	Control 1	Spelling Retardates	Control 2
Perinatal				
Abnormal	11%	14%	17%	10%
Normal (home birth)	27%	21%	24%	15%
Normal (not checked)	16%	27%	19%	20%
Normal (hospital report)	46%	38%	40%	55%
Total number	56	56	42	40

Percentages to the nearest whole number. Chi-square 1 d.f $p > 0.05$

9

Summary and Discussion of the Results of the Psychological and Neurological Examinations and Developmental History

In this chapter are summarized and discussed the results of the psychological and neurological examinations and the developmental history provided by the parents. The summary is in two sections. In the first are indicated separately significant differences between the Reading Retardates and Control 1 and between the Spelling Retardates and Control 2, and in the second, similarities and differences between the Reading and Spelling Retardates.

In Tables 42 and 43 are listed 43 items relating to developmental history (motor, speech and language), the psychological examination which included 11 subtests of the WISC, tests of articulation, sound blending, visual retention, right/left discrimination, finger localization, motor proficiency, handedness, eyedness and footedness, and the neurological examination including tendon reflexes, knee to ankle movements and eye movements. They are arranged in the order of levels of statistical significance.

Summary (Section 1)

Reading Retardates and Control 1

Significant differences between the Reading Retardates and Control 1 were found in 24 of the 43 items, 13 at the 0·1 per cent level, 5 at the 1 per cent level and 6 at the 5 per cent level. Most of the items significant at the 0·1 per cent level reflect speech and language deficits such as defective articulation, noted by parents in early childhood and on examination, low vocabulary score on the WISC, low Verbal IQ and Verbal IQ lower than Performance IQ. Defects are found in the processing of sounds sequentially arranged and requiring reproduction in a precise order either discretely as in digit span or by synthesis as in sound blending. Sequential processes are also involved in the visuo-motor task of coding, which is also poor. Few of the Reading Retardates got beyond the arithmetical questions on the WISC which depend largely on a long-term memory of number combinations and tables. Also highly significant is directional confusion, an inability to discriminate right and left. The test as administered involved a knowledge of right and left, verbal labelling of right and left, and also the ability to hold a sequence of verbal instructions in mind.

Still highly significant, but at the 1 per cent level, is further evidence of late speech development and early language difficulties. The ability to reproduce visually perceived shapes from memory is poor. This weakness is evident both in the smaller number of correctly reproduced designs and in the greater number of errors made.

At the 5 per cent level of significance, differences were found on Block Design, Similarities and on the Test of Motor Proficiency. Delay in walking unaided and early clumsiness are more prevalent among the Reading Retardates. A significantly greater number of boys wrote with the left hand. The results of the test of simultaneous writing indicate further that most of these left-handed writers were not strongly left-handed but ambilateral. Handedness is the only laterality feature which reaches a level of significance among the Reading Retardates. No significant differences were found on 19 items. These include 4 of the WISC subtests, Comprehension, Picture Completion, Picture Arrangement and Object Assembly. When it is recalled that the mean Full Scale IQ of the Control group is 120·0, it is clear that many of these Reading Retardates are performing at quite high levels on some of the functions examined in the intelligence test. Also not significant were the ages at which the earliest motor and speech "milestones" appeared. It would seem that it is not until the more complex activities, using full sentences and walking unaided, are to be expected, that differences become apparent. Apart from very early speech development and the WISC Comprehension subtest, the only test directly involving speech, which did not reach a level of significance. is that of auditory discrimination.

No differences were found with regard to finger localization or those neuromuscular functions tested in the neurological examination.

Spelling Retardates and Control 2

On only 17 of the 43 items listed in Table 43 were significant differences found between the Spelling Retardates and Control 2. Four of these are at the 0·1 per cent level, 3 at the 1 per cent level, and 10 at the 5 per cent level. At the 0·1 per cent level of significance, the Spelling Retardates achieved lower scores on two of the WISC subtests, Digit Span and Coding. Nystagmoid eye movements were found much more frequently, and were more prevalent on deviation to the left than on deviation to the right. At the 1 per cent level of significance were lower scores on the WISC Information subtest, nystagmoid eye movement to the right and fewer boys in whom there was unilateral correspondence of hand, eye and foot.

At the 5 per cent level, were more frequent reports of delayed speech development, early articulatory difficulties and delay in the age at which speech was intelligible. Articulation on examination and the ability to synthesize sounds were poor. Lower scores were obtained in the WISC Arithmetic subtest. A history of early clumsiness was given more frequently and a greater number of Spelling Retardates exhibited an inability to control movement in the Knee to Ankle test. Indeterminate eye-preference and cross-laterality were more prevalent.

No significant differences were found in respect of the earliest speech and motor "milestones," nor were early language difficulties significantly more frequently reported. No differences were found on the WISC IQs or subtests

Table 42
Items relating to the Psychological and Neurological Examinations and
Developmental History ranked by Levels of Significance:
Reading Retardates and Control 1

1. WISC Information	$p < 0.001$
2. WISC Arithmetic	$p < 0.001$
3. Verbal IQ	$p < 0.001$
4. WISC Digit Span	$p < 0.001$
5. Full Scale WISC IQ	$p < 0.001$
6. WISC Coding	$p < 0.001$
7. WISC Vocabulary	$p < 0.001$
8. Right/left discrimination	$p < 0.001$
9. Sound blending	$p < 0.001$
10. Age intelligible speech	$p < 0.001$
11. Early articulatory difficulties	$p < 0.001$
12. Articulation on examination	$p < 0.001$
13. Verbal IQ lower than Performance IQ	$p < 0.001$
14. Age full sentences	$p < 0.01$
15. Early language difficulties	$p < 0.01$
16. Performance IQ	$p < 0.01$
17. Visual retention – number of designs	$p < 0.01$
18. Visual retention – number of errors	$p < 0.01$
19. WISC Similarities	$p < 0.05$
20. WISC Block Design	$p < 0.05$
21. Age walking unaided	$p < 0.05$
22. Motor impairment	$p < 0.05$
23. Early clumsiness	$p < 0.05$
24. Handedness	$p < 0.05$

Not significant:

25. Knee to ankle movement	$p > 0.05$
26. Footedness	$p > 0.05$
27. Hand-eye-foot concordance	$p > 0.05$
28. WISC Object Assembly	$p > 0.05$
29. Age other words	$p > 0.05$
30. Age Mama/Dada	$p > 0.05$
31. WISC Picture Completion	$p > 0.05$
32. WISC Picture Arrangement	$p > 0.05$
33. Cross-laterality	$p > 0.05$
34. Age crawling	$p > 0.05$
35. Age sitting	$p > 0.05$
36. Finger localization	$p > 0.05$
37. Nystagmoid eye movement to right and left	$p > 0.05$
38. Nystagmoid eye movement to right	$p > 0.05$
39. Nystagmoid eye movement to left	$p > 0.05$
40. Tendon reflexes	$p > 0.05$
41. Auditory discrimination	$p > 0.05$
42. WISC Comprehension	$p > 0.05$
43. Eyedness	$p > 0.05$

Table 43

Items relating to the Psychological and Neurological Examinations and
Developmental History ranked by Levels of Significance:
Spelling Retardates and Control 2

1. WISC Digit Span	$p < 0.001$
2. Nystagmoid eye movement to left	$p < 0.001$
3. Nystagmoid eye movement to right and left	$p < 0.001$
4. WISC Coding	$p < 0.001$
5. WISC Information	$p < 0.01$
6. Hand-eye-foot concordance	$p < 0.01$
7. Nystagmoid eye movement to right	$p < 0.01$
8. Cross-laterality	$p < 0.05$
9. Knee to ankle movement	$p < 0.05$
10. Age intelligible speech	$p < 0.05$
11. Early clumsiness	$p < 0.05$
12. Sound blending	$p < 0.05$
13. Early articulatory difficulties	$p < 0.05$
14. Articulation on examination	$p < 0.05$
15. Eyedness	$p < 0.05$
16. WISC Arithmetic	$p < 0.05$
17. Age full sentences	$p < 0.05$

Not significant:

18. Verbal IQ lower than Performance IQ	$p > 0.05$
19. Verbal IQ	$p > 0.05$
20. Age other words	$p > 0.05$
21. WISC Vocabulary	$p > 0.05$
22. Visual retention – number of errors	$p > 0.05$
23. Visual retention – number of design	$p > 0.05$
24. Early language difficulties	$p > 0.05$
25. Full Scale IQ	$p > 0.05$
26. Finger localization	$p > 0.05$
27. Handedness	$p > 0.05$
28. Age Mama/Dada	$p > 0.05$
29. Tendon reflexes	$p > 0.05$
30. Motor impairment	$p > 0.05$
31. Age sitting	$p > 0.05$
32. Age crawling	$p > 0.05$
33. Age walking	$p > 0.05$
34. Auditory discrimination	$p > 0.05$
35. WISC Similarities	$p > 0.05$
36. Right/left discrimination	$p > 0.05$
37. Footedness	$p > 0.05$
*38. Performance IQ	$p > 0.05$
*39. WISC Picture Arrangement	$p > 0.05$
*40. WISC Picture Completion	$p > 0.05$
*41. WISC Comprehension	$p > 0.05$
*42. WISC Block Design	$p > 0.05$
*43. WISC Object Assembly	$p > 0.05$

*Mean scores of Spelling Retardates higher than those of Control 2.

other than the 4 referred to above, nor on the tests of visual retention, right/
left discrimination, finger localization or motor proficiency. Hand and foot
preference did not differentiate the Spelling Retardates from their Controls.

Summary (Section 2)

Similarities and Differences between Reading and Spelling Retardates

The Reading and Spelling Retardates are regarded as similar when both groups
differ significantly from their respective controls. when neither group differs
from its control group or when the difference between one dyslexic group
and its control is not significantly greater than the difference between the
other dyslexic group and its control. The dyslexic groups are regarded as
exhibiting differences when only one of the groups differs from its control
or when a comparison of the differences between each group and its control
reaches a level of statistical significance.

Some of the items listed separately in Tables 42 and 43 are considered
below under a single heading when they clearly relate to similar broad areas of
function. For example, all the activities included in the test of motor proficiency, the tests of eye-movement and of knee to ankle movements involve
voluntary motor control. Likewise handedness, eyedness, footedness, cross-
laterality and hand-eye-foot correspondence are included under the heading
of laterality.

Speech and Language

Both groups include a greater number of boys in whom speech was slow to
develop. The delay was not evident, however, until sentences were used.
There was a higher frequency of early articulatory defects and speech was
later in becoming intelligible. On examination, articulation and the ability to
blend sounds were poor in both groups.

In neither group is comprehension poor, as determined by the WISC. Nor
is there any greater difficulty in perceiving differences between very similar
speech sounds (auditory discrimination).

The groups do differ markedly in the use of language. Early language
difficulties were noted significantly more frequently by parents of the
Reading Retardates. Their poor performance on the WISC vocabulary test
differentiates the Reading Retardates both from their controls and from the
Spelling Retardates. But while only the Reading Retardates differ from their
controls in respect of verbal analogies (Similarities) and the extent to which
Verbal IQ was lower than Performance IQ, on neither of these variables do
they differ significantly from the Spelling Retardates.

Voluntary Motor Control

Common to both groups were significantly more frequent reports by parents
of early clumsiness. Neither group was late in sitting or crawling. But a greater
number of the Reading Retardates were late in walking unaided.

On examination, both groups show some impairment of voluntary motor
co-ordination. In the Reading Retardates, this was most evident on the Test
of Motor Proficiency. Although on the test as a whole, the Spelling Retardates
did not differ significantly from their controls, in both dyslexic groups the
highest failure rate occurred on the tests of balance and manual dexterity.

The incidence of nystagmoid eye movements was high among the Spelling Retardates. They include a greater number of boys whose knee to ankle movements (a test used in the diagnosis of ataxia of the lower limbs) exhibited a lack of smoothness. Although lack of control and inco-ordination of movement is found in both groups, the areas affected differ.

WISC

Both groups obtained significantly lower scores on Information, Arithmetic, Digit Span and Coding, all verbal subtests with the exception of Coding, which is not entirely non-verbal. Neither group differed from their controls on Comprehension, Picture Completion, Picture Arrangement and Object Assembly.

No significant differences were found between Reading and Spelling Retardates on 7 of the 11 subtests. Significant differences were obtained on Information, Arithmetic, Vocabulary and Block Design, the Reading Retardates' scores being lower. Since the Spelling Retardates obtained lower scores than their controls on Information and Arithmetic, the overall pattern of low and high subtest scores is similar in both groups except for Vocabulary and Block Design. The mean Full Scale, Verbal and Performance IQs of the Reading Retardates were lower than those of the Spelling Retardates. However, Verbal-Performance IQ discrepancies were no greater in one group than in the other.

Visual Retention

Although only the Reading Retardates produced a smaller number of correctly reproduced designs and made a greater number of errors than their controls, the differences between Reading and Spelling Retardates were not significant.

Laterality

Atypical patterns of laterality were found with increased frequency in both groups. Among the Reading Retardates the incidence of left-handedness and ambilaterality was higher, whereas among the Spelling Retardates the significant features were eye-preference, cross-laterality and hand-eye-foot correspondence. In neither group do patterns of foot preference differ significantly from controls.

Tendon Reflexes, Finger Localization and Right/Left Discrimination.

In neither group is there a higher incidence of abnormal tendon reflexes or of finger agnosia, but there is a marked difference in respect of right/left discrimination, the Reading Retardates' performance being significantly poorer than that of the Spelling Retardates.

Discussion

In this predominantly middle-class sample of dyslexic boys, there is much evidence of neurodevelopmental delays and anomalies which support the hypothesis that their learning difficulties are constitutional.

The speech and language deficits cannot be explained by low intelligence, lack of opportunity, social deprivation or emotional disturbance. It could be argued that the low WISC Vocabulary and Similarities scores are an effect of the reading retardation and this may be partly so. However, the evidence of late speech development, articulatory defects and early language difficulties suggests that the speech and language delays and deficits precede the reading difficulty. This suggestion is supported by the results of Mason's (1967) inquiry into the reading difficulties experienced by children with early speech disorders. Ingram (1969) has pointed out that in children with a specific retardation of speech development the speech disorders form a continuum. At one end are found delays in the acquisition of word sounds and articulatory difficulties and at the other end speechlessness and a difficulty in comprehension. Clearly the speech difficulties of both dyslexic groups would fall at that end of such a continuum where the disorder is a relatively minor one. It is of interest that the group with the more severe reading disorder has the more extensive speech disorder.

Ingram points out that children with minor speech disorders usually appear normal until they begin to make spontaneous connected utterances. In this study, too, significant delays in the acquisition of speech were not found until the boys reached the age at which sentences were used.

A specific linguistic skill in which both dyslexic groups were deficient is the ability to blend sounds into whole meaningful words. This is an essential skill in reading. A difficulty in synthesizing sounds was thought by Schilder (1944) to be the central feature of reading retardation but it could also be regarded as an effect of the reading retardation. Ingram (1964) and Johnson and Myklebust (1967) included sound-blending difficulties as characteristic of only those dyslexic children with audiophonic difficulties or an auditory dyslexia but not of those whose difficulty related primarily to visuo-spatial deficits. In giving the test of sound blending, the severe difficulty of some children, including a few who could read, was striking. They appeared unable to appreciate that a word could be separated into smaller units of sound or that such sounds could be blended into familiar whole words. It was as if words existed only as single unanalysable sound patterns. Although poor performance on blending sounds could be partly an effect of the reading difficulty, the presence of other speech and language disorders from an early age favours the view that a difficulty in sound blending is another aspect of a developmental language disability.

The test of motor-co-ordination revealed evidence of neurological dysfunction. In both dyslexic groups there was a significant excess of boys who had shown signs of early clumsiness. In both groups there was also, on examination, a greater number of boys with poor voluntary motor control, although different areas of movement were affected.

Abnormalities of motor function in specifically retarded readers were observed by Orton (1937) and more recently by Lovell and Gorton (1968) and by Rutter, Tizard and Whitmore (1970). In this study, a more general clumsiness is found in the presence of a severe reading retardation and a more specific dysfunction of knee to ankle and eye-movement in the presence of a lesser degree of reading difficulty.

Another neurological finding was the greater frequency of atypical laterality patterns. Ambilaterality distinguishes the Reading Retardates both from other Centre boys and from their controls and this is true of the higher incidence of cross-laterality among the Spelling Retardates.

The high incidence of ambilaterality among the Reading Retardates suggests that, in some at least, cerebral dominance is not fully established. Although the relationship between the dominant cerebral hemisphere, that which subserves language, and the dominant hand is now known to be not so direct as Orton (1937) thought, there is evidence that in the left-handed, the ambilateral and those with left-handed relatives, left cerebral dominance is less likely to be fully established than in the fully right-handed (Zangwill, 1960, 1962 b; Milner *et al.,* 1964). The EEG recordings from a group of severely dyslexic children with a high proportion of left-handedness and ambilaterality were consistent with delayed or incomplete cerebral dominance (Newton, 1970). Delay or disturbance of function such as slow speech development, defects in drawing and copying, a weakness in spatial orientation and right/left confusion have been noted in left-handed and more particularly ambilateral children (Zangwill, 1960; Naidoo, 1961). Zangwill has suggested some reasons why only a minority of left-handed or ambilateral children exhibit such disturbances (see page 15). In this sample not all left-handed or ambilateral boys were, for example, late in acquiring speech, but of the 9 who were very late in using sentences, 6 were either left-handed or ambilateral or had a left-handed close relative. Incomplete or delayed cerebral dominance would seem to be one factor contributing to the severe reading backwardness shown by some Reading Retardates.

The atypical patterns of laterality found among the Spelling Retardates are mixed eye-preference and cross-laterality. The significance of cross-laterality is obscure. The increased frequency of nystagmoid eye movements among the Spelling Retardates raises the possibility that these, in some way not understood, may influence eye preference. Should this be so, then there may be two types of cross-laterality, one associated with a minor ocular neuromuscular weakness, the other not so associated. Of the 14 boys exhibiting a nystagmoid movement, 10 were cross-lateral.

Of the four WISC subtests on which both dyslexic groups obtained significantly lower scores than their respective controls, two, Digit Span and Coding, are unlikely to be an effect of the reading retardation. The results of these subtests are in keeping with the findings of others (Altus, 1956; Lovell, Shapton and Warren, 1964; Belmont and Birch, 1966; Reid and Schoer, 1966; and Doehring, 1968). Milner's work (1962) with adults who had sustained a lesion or excision of the left temporal lobe, has shown that where the left cerebral hemisphere is dominant for language there is regularly a selective impairment in the recall of verbal material. One cannot infer brain damage in children who show a selective impairment of immediate auditory recall, but it would seem reasonable to suggest that in some children a specific and severe deficit of this kind reflects a neurological dysfunction or delay In the remedial teaching situation at the Centre, children with very low scores on Digit Span invariably gave evidence of a more general difficulty in the recall of verbal material and such children were found extremely difficult to teach, their progress being inordinately slow.

So many backward readers, not only those with a specific reading disability, perform poorly on the WISC Coding subtest, that the low scores obtained by both dyslexic groups may be without especial significance. Although classified as a Performance subtest, the test involves verbal, visual and motor functions. Scores are less often low because of errors made in inscribing the appropriate symbol than because of slow performance. Visual perceptual and motor speed are required since the test is timed and these are skills in which the specifically retarded reader seems deficient (Doehring, 1968). The tests of Manual Dexterity included in the test of motor pro- ficiency are also timed and failure was often recorded because the tasks were not completed in the allotted time. The high failure rate in both dyslexic groups on the test of manual dexterity and the low coding scores may have been partly due to a slowness in executing a motor response

Further evidence of developmental delay comes from the significantly lower scores of the Reading Retardates on the test of right/left discrimination, in keeping with other reports (Hermann, 1959; Belmont and Birch, 1965; Rutter, Tizard and Whitmore, 1970). Every effort was made in administering this test to minimize confusions due to faulty verbal labelling or to a difficulty in remembering the verbal instructions which were quite lengthy in some items. There is little doubt that none the less linguistic factors accounted for some failures. Benton (1958) has stressed the dependency of right/left discri- mination.on language. It is noteworthy that in this study, right-left confusion is marked only among the Reading Retardates in whom there is evidence of quite extensive speech and language difficulties. The results of the Cluster Analysis (see Chapter 11) are of further relevance to the question of the extent to which right-left confusions may be associated with language difficulties.

On the test of visual retention, the Reading Retardates obtained poorer scores than their controls on the number of correct designs and on the number of errors. When chronological age and Full Scale IQ were taken into account to determine whether or not performance was commensurate with an expected level, no difference was found. This would indicate that a *specific* visual memory or visuo-motor defect was not more common among the Reading Retardates. The marked discrepancy between the WISC subtest scaled scores raises another possibility. Where marked discrepancies are found, and these are common among dyslexic children, the reliability of the Full Scale IQ as an indicator of the level of intelligence is doubtful. It is possible that in such cases the use of the Full Scale IQ in evaluating scores may produce a misleading conclusion about whether or not performance on the test of visual retention is within normal limits.

The differences, found in both groups on the WISC Arithmetic subtest, could be interpreted as reflecting a learning difficulty unrelated to the reading difficulty, or as arising from a deficit which underlies both the arithmetic and the reading difficulty, or as an effect of the reading difficulty. In the test reading is required only in the last three problems and few dyslexic boys reached this point. At school children are required to read the questions. If they cannot read or read inaccurately they may become confused about arith- metic. Errors on the test can be due either to an unreliable knowledge of number combinations and tables or to a failure to understand and/or to compute the problems correctly or to a combination of these. The rote learning of number combinations and tables involves the learning of three numbers in association, such as four plus seven is eleven, three times six is eighteen. Sequential learning is essential and the application of these "rules" is carried out under conditions of long-term recall. The understanding and computation of problems depends upon an ability to form verbal concepts which allow no margin for imprecision. Difficulties in carrying out these processes could underlie a difficulty both to calculate and to read.

One negative finding deserves comment. On the test of auditory discrimination, no difference was found between either dyslexic group and its control group. In this middle-class sample, the standard of articulation as well as of language in the home, is likely to be high. This raises the question of whether where significant differences have been found, it is the quality of speech in the environment which has been the main contributory factor. Another reason for our negative finding may be the rigorous exclusion of boys with a hearing loss, however slight.

Both groups of dyslexic boys of at least average intelligence, give evidence of disorders of a neurophysiological nature, particularly the speech and language delays, the motor dysfunctions and the atypical patterns of laterality present from an early age. It is noteworthy that so many findings from this study should be similar to those from a recent total population survey (Rutter, Tizard and Whitmore, 1970). The importance of neuro-developmental disorders is amply demonstrated and supports the contention that dyslexia has a constitutional basis. There is no evidence to suggest that, in a significant proportion of these dyslexics, the disorders are acquired as the result of perinatal trauma or other pre- or perinatal factors. But the higher, although statistically insignificant, incidence of some of these among the dyslexics suggests that the possibility of an acquired disorder cannot be ruled out in some cases. Whether these developmental reading disorders might be genetically determined is considered in the following chapter.

The delays and disabilities found in both groups of dyslexics and the many areas in which no differences were found between them support the hypothesis that their disorders are of an essentially similar nature. The higher levels of the significance of the differences between the Reading Retardates and their controls and the more extensive dysfunctions found among Reading Retardates suggest that a severe disability is more likely to be associated with a wider range of developmental anomaly that a less severe one. The more severe dyslexia is also associated with lower Verbal, Performance and Full Scale IQs. In view of the marked subtest discrepancies, the value of a composite IQ as a reliable indicator of intelligence must be questioned. Both the early speech and language disorders and the reading difficulty itself are likely, at least partly, to contribute to the level of "intelligence" as expressed by the IQ. Children who cannot read are debarred from the extensive reading which improves vocabulary and the use of language.

Not all the dyslexic boys exhibited delays or impairment in all areas of function. The only defects common to all were the reading and spelling difficulties. The question of whether other defects were associated with each other so as to form different types of dyslexia was explored by the cluster analysis reported in Chapter 11.

10

Reading, Spelling and Speech Difficulties and Left-handedness in Other Members of the Family

The main reason for regarding specific dyslexia as a familial disorder is the frequency with which a family history of reading difficulty is reported. The reliability of histories is variable. At best, such histories are only suggestive of genetic determination. Difficulties may or may not have been specific, and may be due to a number of reasons. In this study, information was obtained from the parents about the presence or previous history of reading and spelling difficulties, speech difficulties and left-handedness, wholly or partial, in parents and siblings only. Additional information volunteered suggests that these difficulties were often present in other more distant relatives.

Family History of Reading and Spelling Difficulties

Both a delay in learning to read and severe and persisting reading difficulty are included under "reading difficulty." A positive history in one or more members of the family was given for 32·7 per cent of the Reading Retardates, 14·5 per cent of Control 1 ($p < 0.05$), 42·1 per cent of the Spelling Retardates and 7·5 per cent of Control 2 ($p < 0.001$).

Sixteen fathers had some reading difficulty (6 Reading, 9 Spelling Retardates, 1 Control 1). The difference between the Spelling Retardates and Control 2 is significant ($p < 0.01$). Twelve mothers had experienced a reading difficulty (4 Reading, 6 Spelling Retardates, 1 Control 1, 1 Control 2). In four families both parents were affected (1 Reading, 3 Spelling Retardates).

The number of siblings with reading difficulties was not recorded but only whether affected siblings were male or female. Of the 57 dyslexics with brothers, 15 had at least one brother experiencing some reading difficulty. A similar number of the Control boys had brothers but in only 4 of these families was a reading difficulty experienced by at least one brother. Sixty dyslexics had sisters, a reading difficulty occurring in the female siblings of five such families but in only 2 of the 57 controls with sisters.

While a spelling difficulty almost invariably accompanied a reading difficulty, poor spelling in other members of the family was reported more frequently than a reading difficulty. The percentages of families with a history of spelling difficulties were 53·8 per cent Reading Retardates, 16·4 per cent Control 1 ($p < 0.001$), 56·4 per cent Spelling Retardates and 7·5 per cent Control 2 ($p < 0.001$).

Table 44
Family History of Reading and Spelling Difficulties

Family history	Reading Retardates	Control 1	Spelling Retardates	Control 2
Reading difficulty	32·7%	14·5%*	42·1%	7·5%***
No reading difficulty	67·3%	85·5%	57·9%	92·5%
Total number	52	55	38	40
Spelling difficulty	53·8%	16·4%***	56·4%	7·5%***
No spelling difficulty	46·2%	83·6%	43·6%	92·5%
Total number	52	55	39	40

Chi-square 1 d.f.
   *Significant at 5% level.
***Significant at 0·1% level.

Familial Reading and/or Spelling Difficulties in the Control Groups
In the control groups combined, 4 were reading 2 years or more below chronological age and a further 3 had a specific spelling difficulty, reading above chronological age level but retarded in spelling by 2 years or more. In 3 of the 7 boys (42·8 per cent) there was a history of reading or spelling difficulty. The numbers are too small to draw any conclusion but the proportion is noteworthy for its similarity to that found among the dyslexics.

Familial Speech Difficulties
The difficulties were those of speech, such as articulatory defects, stammering and stuttering and not of language. Altogether such speech difficulties were reported in 23 families (those of 7 Reading, 8 Spelling Retardates, 5 Control 1 and 3 Control 2). The difference in frequency between each dyslexic group and its control is not significant.

   In six families the father was said to have some speech disorder (2 Reading, 2 Spelling Retardates and 2 Control 2) and in three families it was the mother (Spelling Retardates). While brothers of 15 dyslexics had a speech difficulty this was reported for brothers of only 2 control boys. The subjects who had sisters with a speech disorder were more evenly distributed (7 dyslexic, 5 control).

   There appears to be some preponderance of familial speech difficulties among male members of the families of the dyslexics which is not found among the controls.

Table 45
Speech Difficulty in Family

	Reading Retardates	Control 1	Spelling Retardates	Control 2
Speech Difficulty				
Yes	13·5%	9·1%	21·1%	7·5%
No	86·5%	90·9%	78·9%	92·5%
Total number	52	55	38	40

Chi-square 1 d.f. $p > 0.05$

Familial Left-handedness

In completing the Family Information Questionnaire, left-handedness and mixed laterality were both recorded for the same person in a few cases. Since the parents of the control boys were not interviewed this could not be checked. In Table 46 left-handedness includes those who are left-handed and/or ambilateral, that is those wholly or partially left-handed.

While there is a greater number of boys in both dyslexic groups whose families included one or more members who were wholly or partially left-handed, no significant differences were found between each dyslexic group and its control (42·3 per cent Reading, 50 per cent Spelling Retardates, 29·1 per cent Control 1 and 35 per cent Control 2). The highest frequency of familial left-handedness or ambilaterality is found among the Spelling Retardates.

Table 46
Left-handedness in Family

	Reading Retardates	Control 1	Spelling Retardates	Control 2
Left-handed/Mixed Laterality				
Yes	42·3%	29·1%	50·0%	35·0%
No	57·7%	70·9%	50·0%	65·0%
Total number	52	55	36	40

Chi-square 1 d.f. $p > 0.05$

Discussion

In both groups combined, 36·7 per cent of the dyslexic boys had a family history of reading difficulty, compared with 11·5 per cent of all controls. These percentages are remarkably similar to those found in the Isle of Wight Survey in which a family history was reported in 33·7 per cent of children with a specific reading retardation and in 9·2 per cent of the controls (Rutter. Tizard and Whitmore, 1970). That survey also found a higher frequency (41·2 per cent) among the specifically retarded readers who were not maladjusted, compared with the 20·7 per cent among those who were maladjusted specifically retarded readers. In this study, boys considered to be severely maladjusted were excluded. The incidence of family histories of reading difficulty is higher among the Spelling Retardates (42·1 per cent) than among the Reading Retardates (32·7 per cent). It was seen in the section in Behaviour in School (Chapter 6) that a greater number of Reading than of Spelling Retardates were classified as "unsettled" on the Bristol Social Adjustment Guide. This could be an effect of the more severe nature of the learning difficulty among the Reading Retardates. It is also possible that the Reading Retardates tended to be less stable and that this factor might contribute to the *degree* of the reading failure.

Reading difficulties were reported more frequently in male than in female relatives, particularly among the dyslexics. Since the number of the boys' siblings was not recorded, a comparison could not be made between the number of male and female relatives with a positive history.

It was fully expected that, in this clinic sample of dyslexic boys, an unusually high proportion would give a positive family history of reading difficulty. But their similarity to the percentages found in the Isle of Wight Survey is remarkable. Among the control boys with a specific reading disability, admittedly few in number, the proportion with a positive family history is again strikingly similar.

In a considerable number of dyslexic boys a genetic aetiology is strongly suggested and the constancy of the proportion is noteworthy.

Summary

A family history of reading, spelling and speech difficulties and some degree of left-handedness are found more commonly in both dyslexic groups, but differences in frequency reach levels of significance only with regard to reading and spelling difficulties. A family history of reading difficulty was found in 36·7 per cent of all dyslexics and in 11·5 per cent of all controls, percentages which are very similar to those of the specifically retarded readers (33·7 per cent) and the controls (9·2 per cent) in the Isle of Wight Survey (Rutter, Tizard and Whitmore, 1970).

11

One Disorder or Many ?

Introduction: Aims of the Cluster Analysis

Many features indicative of developmental delay have been found to distinguish the dyslexics from their controls. But only the specific reading and spelling retardation is common to all. The finding that there is no other defect in all these dyslexics is in keeping with the results of previous investigations.

Experience both in examining and in teaching dyslexic children suggests that certain deficits are associated with each other so as to form distinctive patterns of disability and the hypothesis has been advanced that there are sub-groups or types of dyslexia resulting from or associated with different underlying learning difficulties (Ingram, 1964; Johnson and Myklebust, 1967). One type is thought to be characterized by speech and language disorders, the dyslexia probably being a residuum of slow language learning (Mason, 1967). Another appears to be associated with visuo-spatial deficits. The issues involved are not only of theoretical importance but crucial to the planning of appropriate remedial programmes.

Distinctions on the basis of differing aetiology have also been made, between dyslexics in whom the disorder seems to be genetically determined and those in whom the dyslexia is symptomatic of early brain injury. The term "specific dyslexia" is most frequently applied only to the former category (Critchley, 1964). In practice it is often very difficult if not impossible to make such distinctions.

In this study there were recorded the presence or absence of reading and of spelling difficulties in parents and siblings only, since information about other affected relatives was likely to vary from family to family. In some cases, although there was no positive history in the immediate family, this was reported in more distant relatives. But there are also many boys in this sample whose parents, after exhaustive inquiry, could report no affected relative. Many dyslexic boys, although showing no gross defect on neurological examination, exhibited minor abnormalities which raise the question of whether their reading difficulties are acquired. Evidence of perinatal complications would strengthen the possibility that early brain injury might have been sustained.

The possibility was explored that there may be within this sample more than one type of dyslexia, distinguishable by different configurations of

98

associated impairment, by submitting to a cluster analysis data from the
psychological examination, from the developmental histories and from the
neurological examination. By adding data on family histories of reading, of
spelling and of speech difficulties and of left-handedness and on perinatal
history, an attempt is made to discover whether different patterns of disability might be associated with different aetiological factors.

Cluster Analysis, Procedures

On the suggestion of Mr. Harvey Goldstein, a programme developed by the
Rothamsted Experimental Station was used, which would accept data both
quantitative and qualitative. Essentially the procedures employed enable the
investigator to detect the presence or absence of relationships between multi-
dimensional configurations. Each variable is given equal weight. For a pair of
boys, a similarity coefficient is calculated which varies between 0 and 1, so
that if there is complete agreement on the values of all the variables measured
the similarity is 1, and if no agreement the similarity is 0. These coefficients
are computed for each pair of boys and every boy has a set of similarity
coefficients, one with every other boy. All the information required for the
single linkage cluster analysis is contained in the Minimum Spanning Tree
(MST). In the representation of the MST, all boys (points) are joined by
lines associated with the "distance" between them. This "distance" is
inversely related to the similarity - the greater the similarity the shorter the
distance. Each boy represented on the MST is linked to his closest neighbour,
i.e. that boy with whom the similarity coefficient is highest. If all lines above
a given distance are severed, this leaves "clusters" of boys all joined together
by links, each less than this distance. This given distance is open to choice.
The single linkage cluster analysis can be performed by including the links of
a Minimum Spanning Tree in decreasing order of size. Decreasing the distance
by gradual steps results in a hierarchical sequence of splitting clusters. If
"natural" clusters do not emerge, the MST can provide artificial clusters by
removing suitable links, although individuals very similar to others may then
be in neighbouring clusters instead of in one. Unlike a multi-variate analysis,
the single linkage cluster analysis does not have a probabilistic basis. No
hypotheses are tested although, as in this case, specific hypotheses may
determine which variables are to be submitted to the cluster analysis. In the
event of clusters emerging, hypotheses relating to the composition of these
can be examined by conventional statistical techniques. The explanation of
the procedures involved is simplified and for fuller details the reader is
referred to the description given by Gower and Ross (1969).

The variables listed below were selected, these relating to developmental
history, neurological status, speech, language, auditory memory, visuo-spatial
function, arithmetic, perinatal status, and familial factors (reading, spelling,
speech and left-handedness).

The cluster analysis was carried out on both groups of dyslexics combined.
The first run-through of the programme revealed that lack of information
about many of the variables in four cases created an artificial bias, so these
were dropped from subsequent computations. The following results concern
94 boys only.

Severing the MST at several distance thresholds was tried in an attempt to
identify clusters without any clear clusters emerging. Instead there appeared

Variables Submitted to Cluster Analysis

Developmental history	(a) age walking unaided
	(b) age words used
	(c) age pronunciation clear
Speech and language	(a) articulation – score
	(b) auditory discrimination – score
	(c) sound blending – score
	(d) WISC Comprehension – scaled score
	(e) WISC Similarities – scaled score
	(f) WISC Vocabulary – scaled score
Immediate auditory recall	WISC Digit Span – scaled score
Visuo-spatial	(a) WISC Picture Completion – scaled score
	(b) WISC Picture Arrangement – scaled score
	(c) WISC Block Design – scaled score
	(d) WISC Object Assembly – scaled score
Visual recall	Visual Retention Test
	(a) designs – Number of points below the norm for CA and IQ
	(b) errors – Number of points above the norm for CA and IQ
Arithmetic	WISC Arithmetic – scaled score
Laterality	Handedness on Simultaneous Writing
	Footedness
	Cross-laterality
	Hand-eye-foot concordance
Right/left discrimination	Test score
Neurological	(a) tendon reflexes
	(b) knee to ankle test
	(c) eye movements
	(d) motor impairment score
	(e) finger localization
Social adjustment	Bristol Social Adjustment Guide – total score
Perinatal status	Physician's assessment
Familial factors	(a) reading difficulties – mother, father, sisters, brothers
	(b) spelling difficulties – mother, father, sisters, brothers
	(c) speech difficulties – mother, father, sisters, brothers
	(d) left-handedness – complete or partial – mother, father, sisters, brothers.

to be a continuum. At a distance threshold of 18·5, five groups could be identified, containing 27, 5, 3, 3 and 2 boys. The largest group extended along the centre of the MST, while the remaining very small groups were found at one extreme end. Above this distance threshold, the groups amalgamated. Below it a large group at the "core" of the MST was still evident and a greater number of very small groups. An examination of the variables in each of the groups emerging at the distance threshold of 18·5, revealed that only 2 of the boys in the only large group had relatives with a reading difficulty while 11 of the 13 boys in the four small groups gave a positive family history. Boys with a positive family history seemed to be more numerous at one end of

the MST. Only 3 of the 13 boys gave an abnormal response on the neurological tests in contrast to 11 of the 27 in the large group. Most of the latter
were found at the opposite end of the MST. It seemed possible that the
continuum apparent in the MST might be characterized by a predominance
of "genetic" dyslexics at one extreme, a predominance of dyslexics with a
minor neurological dysfunction at the other extreme and perhaps boys with
both of these features at the centre. All boys, that is points, on the MST with
familial reading and spelling difficulties and those giving some abnormal
neurological response were identified. But although boys with a positive
family history and no abnormal neurological response were mostly found at
one end of the MST, the continuum suggested above was not clearly evident.

It seemed worth while however to investigate some groups further. By
removing three links on the MST, four groups were created. The decision to
remove these particular links was made on the hypothesis that a genetic
dyslexia could be distinguished from one possibly acquired and associated
with minor neurological dysfunction. The separation of close neighbours on
the MST was avoided.

Group 1 comprises 20 of the 27 boys in the large group emerging
"naturally" at the distance threshold of 18·5. Group 2 includes 33 boys at
one end of the MST. Group 3 comprises 6 boys. They include 5 of the 15
boys giving an abnormal response on some part of the neurological examination without also having a family history of reading or spelling difficulty.
Group 4 also includes 6 boys, in 4 of whom the neurological examination was
not entirely negative and who also give a positive family history. The
Minimum Spanning Tree showing the position of boys with possible minimal
neurological dysfunction and/or a positive family history, and Groups 1, 2,
3 and 4 is displayed on page 102.

Since these groups were artificially created, since the distances vary
between as well as within the groups and since the numbers differ so
markedly, hypotheses relating to characteristics which might distinguish one
group from another could not reasonably be tested statistically. It was hoped
instead that by examining the frequency with which disorders occurred in
these groups, tentative hypotheses might be formulated relating to patterns
of disability associated with different aetiological factors.

In Group 1, there is an equal number, 10, of Reading and of Spelling
Retardates and in Group 2, 22 Reading and 11 Spelling Retardates. Group 3
contains only Reading Retardates and Group 4, 2 Reading and 4 Spelling
Retardates. Reading and Spelling Retardates are found in all groups except
Group 3. The mean ages of boys in the four groups are very similar, 121·1,
121·6, 121·5 and 120·0 months in Groups 1, 2, 3 and 4 respectively.

Results

Wherever possible, frequencies rather than means have been calculated.
Specific criteria have been employed which would indicate a delay or
response other than that which might normally be expected. This does not
mean that a response which fails to meet a given criterion is abnormal but
merely that it is atypical or reflects some difficulty. In addition to giving the
means of the WISC subtest scaled scores, the frequency of scaled scores
falling below the standardization mean (10) minus one standard deviation

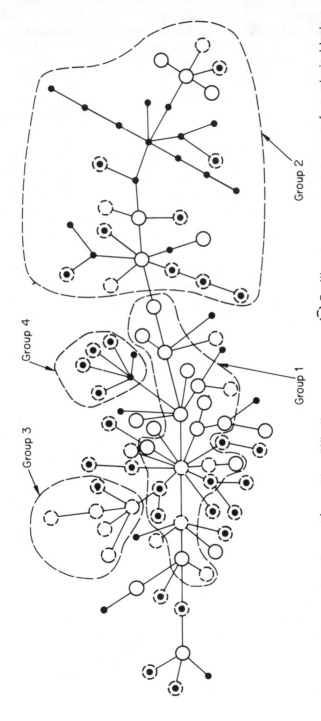

● Family history of reading and/or spelling difficulty ⟨◌⟩ Positive response on one or more of neurological tests

Fig. 3
Minimum Spanning Tree — 94 dyslexic boys

Table 4.7

Cluster Analysis: Number of Boys in Groups 1, 2, 3 and 4 and Percentage showing Response or history as indicated in Table against each Variable

	Group 1 (20) Mean age 121.1 mths		Group 2 (33) Mean age 121.6 mths		Group 3 (6) Mean age 121.5 mths		Group 4 (6) Mean age 120.0 mths	
1. Walking unaided – 18 months or later	20	10%	26	12%	5	40%	6	17%
2. Words used – 13 months or later	15	7%	15	60%	2	0%	4	0%
3. Age pronunciation clear – 4 years or later	16	13%	20	50%	5	40%	5	20%
4. Present articulation not clear – score ≤ 96	19	32%	28	29%	5	40%	6	17%
5. Auditory discrimination difficulty – ≤ 5 errors	20	10%	32	25%	6	17%	6	33%
6. Sound blending – score < 4	20	65%	32	6%	6	100%	6	50%
7. WISC Comprehension — S.S. ≤ 6	20	0%	32	0%	6	0%	6	0%
8. WISC Similarities — S.S. ≤ 6	20	0%	32	3%	6	0%	6	0%
9. WISC Vocabulary — S.S. ≤ 6	20	0%	31	0%	6	0%	6	0%
10. WISC Digit span — S.S. ≤ 6	20	0%	31	39%	6	67%	5	0%
11. WISC Picture Completion — S.S. ≤ 6	20	0%	30	0%	6	0%	6	0%
12. WISC Picture Arrangement — S.S. ≤ 6	20	0%	32	0%	6	17%	6	17%
13. WISC Block Design — S.S. ≤ 6	20	0%	32	0%	6	0%	6	0%
14. WISC Object Assembly — S.S. ≤ 6	20	0%	32	0%	6	17%	6	17%
15. WISC Coding — S.S. ≤ 5	20	15%	32	9%	6	17%	6	0%
16. Visual retention – outside norm for CA & IQ	20	10%	33	21%	6	67%	6	17%
17. WISC Arithmetic — S.S. ≤ 6	19	10%	32	12%	6	83%	6	0%
18. Handedness – left or ambilateral	20	40%	31	19%	6	67%	6	33%
19. Footedness – left or indeterminate	20	65%	31	42%	6	83%	5	100%
20. Cross-lateral	20	70%	31	45%	6	83%	6	33%
21. Hand/eye/foot non-correspondence	20	95%	31	58%	6	100%	6	100%
22. Right/left confusion – score ≤ 15	20	35%	29	41%	6	17%	6	17%
23. Social Adjustment, 'unstable' (BSAG score 16–19)	20	15%	33	15%	6	33%	6	50%
24. Tendon reflexes – other than normal	19	21%	30	17%	6	83%	6	17%
25. Knee to Ankle movement – other than normal	16	13%	25	28%	4	75%	6	33%
26. Nystagmoid eye movement	15	27%	23	17%	5	60%	6	33%
27. Abnormal response on 24, 25 or 26	20	40%	30	40%	6	100%	6	67%
28. Motor impairment – score ≤ 5	19	16%	32	19%	6	17%	6	17%
29. Finger Localization – performance at 5th percentile or below	20	5%	30	20%	6	0%	6	0%
30. Perinatal abnormal	20	10%	33	9%	6	67%	6	0%
31. Reading difficulty in other member of family	20	5%	31	52%	6	17%	5	80%
32. Spelling difficulty in other member of family	23	10%	31	71%	6	0%	6	100%
33. Speech difficulty in other member of family	20	5%	30	27%	6	0%	6	17%
34. Left-handedness in other member of family	20	30%	31	52%	6	17%	6	100%

First column for each group represents total number of boys for whom relevant item of information obtained. Percentages to nearest whole number.

(3), that is, scaled scores of 6 or less, has been calculated. It will be recalled that all boys are of at least average intelligence. The frequencies have been converted to percentages and these with the WISC subtest means and Intelligence Quotients are given in Tables 47 and 48.

Table 48
Cluster Analysis: Mean WISC Subtest Scaled Scores, Verbal IQ and Performance IQ in Groups 1, 2, 3 and 4

	Group 1 (20)	Group 2 (33)	Group 3 (6)	Group 4 (6)
Comprehension	13·0	11·8	11·0	11·8
Arithmetic	9·4	10·2	6·0	10·9
Similarities	12·5	12·9	12·0	11·8
Vocabulary	13·2	11·6	12·5	13·0
Digit Span	9·1	8·3	6·5	8·8
Picture Completion	12·8	12·8	10·5	10·1
Picture Arrangement	11·4	10·7	8·9	9·9
Block Design	13·7	13·1	10·7	12·1
Object Assembly	12·3	13·0	8·7	10·5
Coding	10·1	10·6	8·3	9·1
Verbal IQ	111·9	108·2	98·6	109·7
Performance IQ	115·0	113·4	96·5	105·5

Family History
The percentage of boys with family histories of reading, spelling and speech difficulties and of left-handedness is considerably higher in Groups 2 and 4 than in either Group 1 or 3. Group 2 has the highest incidence of familial speech difficulty while every boy in Group 3 has a left-handed relative. Since inquiries were restricted to the boys' parents and siblings, it is possible that boys in all groups may have other relatives with reading, spelling or speech difficulties, or be left-handed. A positive family history, while suggesting a genetic aetiology, by no means proves it. But it would seem that if the learning disorder in any of the four groups is genetically determined, the likelihood is greater in Groups 2 and 4.

Perinatal History and Neurological Findings
It is not claimed that the variations found in the tendon reflexes, the knee to ankle movement or the eye movements are evidence of neurological damage or even dysfunction when occurring in isolation among otherwise normal children. Of the boys who exhibited any one of these signs between 66 and 75 per cent of the boys in Groups 1, 2 and 4 exhibited only one. But in Group 3 each boy gave an abnormal response and in 4 of the 6 boys two or all three responses were positive. Four of the 6 boys had an abnormal perinatal history, a higher proportion than was found in any other group. Two of these, one delivered by forceps and another slightly asphyxiated, had given no reason for anxiety at the time of birth.

WISC
Differences between Verbal and Performance IQ and between the subtest scores provide information about relative abilities and disabilities. In each of the four groups, differences between mean Verbal and Performance IQ are

not great but the direction of the difference is of interest. Both Groups 1 and 2 show a tendency towards a negative discrepancy, the mean Verbal IQ being lower than Performance IQ. In Groups 3 and 4 this tendency is reversed.

Bannatyne (1966) has suggested that the "genetic" dyslexic would show low verbal and high spatial ability and that children with a minimal neurological dysfunction would show high verbal and low spatial ability. He suggested that the genetic dyslexic especially would perform poorly on the subtests involving sequencing abilities. Bannatyne divided the WISC subtests into three categories relating to Verbal Conceptualizing Ability (Comprehension, Similarities and Vocabulary), Spatial Ability (Picture Completion, Block Design and Object Assembly) and Sequencing Ability (Digit Span, Picture Arrangement and Coding).

The mean scaled scores for these three categories are given in Table 49 (the score falling at the 50th percentile is 30 in each category).

Table 49

Mean Scaled Scores for Verbal Conceptualizing Ability, Spatial Ability and Sequencing Ability, Groups 1, 2, 3 and 4

	Group 1 Mean	Group 2 Mean	Group 3 Mean	Group 4 Mean
Verbal Conceptualizing Ability	38·7	35·9	34·2	36·7
Spatial Ability	38·9	38·1	29·7	33·9
Sequencing Ability	30·7	29·4	23·7	26·3

While the direction of the differences between the means supports Bannatyne's hypothesis that Verbal scores are lower than Spatial scores in the "genetic" group, Group 2, and that Spatial scores are lower than Verbal scores in the "neurological" group, Group 3, the differences between Verbal and Spatial scores are not great. This rearrangement of the subtests does emphasize however, the relatively poor performance by *all four* groups on the tests of sequencing ability.

The mean Verbal IQ for Group 3 is 98·6. But their scores on the subtests of Verbal Conceptualizing Ability shows that their verbal ability is not as far below that of the other groups as the Verbal IQ might suggest.

Group 1 (20 boys) is remarkable for the rarity of reading, spelling and speech difficulties in the immediate family. The incidence of familial left-handedness is no higher than in the control groups. Yet 1 boy out of 4 was strongly left-handed. Two boys out of 3 were cross-lateral and 2 out of 3 of indeterminate footedness. In 19 of the 20, unilateral preference of hand, eye and foot were not concordant. One out of 3 boys showed a marked right/left confusion, and in 5 out of 7 this was associated with cross-laterality or indeterminate footedness. Articulation was poor but not defective in 6 out of 19 of boys. Ignoring atypical patterns of laterality and low sound blending scores, both common in this group, only 4 boys gave no evidence of delay or deficit on some part of the psychological or neurological examination. In the majority, as the low percentages in Table 47 might suggest, only one or two isolated features were found in each case, there being no discernible pattern of association between deficits. On the basis of the total scores on the Bristol Social Adjustment Guide, this is a very "stable" group.

Group 2 (33 boys) is labelled a "genetic" group. Of 31 boys, 24 had a close relative with reading and/or spelling difficulty. In 13 of these, at least 2 other members of the family were affected. Information was missing in 2 cases. The incidence of familial speech difficulties is highest in this group. Precise information about early speech development was not given for many boys in all groups. But where this was recorded, delays are found more frequently among the boys in Group 2 than in any other group. Late speech development, a delay in speech becoming intelligible, poor articulation or defective auditory discrimination were found in 24 boys, 72·7 per cent, the percentages in the other groups being 45 per cent in Group 1, 50 per cent in Group 3 and 33·3 per cent in Group 4. Right/left confusion is more prevalent in Group 2 and is associated most frequently with speech or language delays or defects. Apart from one boy in Group 1, finger agnosia was found only in Group 2. In only 3 of the 6 boys, who had difficulty in localizing the position of their fingers, was there also a right/left confusion and a marked difficulty on the WISC Arithmetic subtest, suggestive of a developmental Gerstmann syndrome. The frequency of each aspect of laterality examined approximated closely to that found among the control groups, although the incidence of familial left-handedness is higher than in any group except 4.

Group 3 (6 boys). One boy had a family history of reading difficulty and another a left-handed relative. The perinatal history was abnormal in four. Each of the 6 gave an abnormal response to some part of the neurological examination, involving tendon reflexes in 5, knee to ankle movements in 3 and eye movements in 3. No boy achieved a score of less than 2 and one had a high impairment score on the test of motor proficiency. Two of 5 were late in walking unaided. Unfortunately precise information about early speech development was available for 2 boys only, neither of whom showed any delay. Verbal conceptualizing ability is of a higher order than spatial ability. Marked deficits in immediate auditory recall and in arithmetic were more common in this group than in any other. In each boy the WISC subtest scaled scores are widely discrepant. Despite the use of the Full Scale IQ in determining whether performance was at or below an expected level, 4 of the 6 boys gave evidence of a specific visuo-motor or visual retention deficit. Although only 1 boy had a left-handed close relative, the incidence of left-handedness or ambilaterality is highest in this group.

Group 4 (6 boys) would seem to be another "genetic" group but they present a marked contrast in some respects to Group 2. While familial speech difficulties are more frequent in Group 2, each boy in the present Group has at least 1 left-handed relative. Only 1 boy was strongly left-handed and another ambilateral, but foot preferences in each is indeterminate. Spatial ability is lower than verbal ability. The WISC Arithmetic mean is highest and no boy showed a marked difficulty. Three of the 6 boys were "unstable" according to the Bristol Social Adjustment Guide, the highest proportion found in any group. No boy had an abnormal perinatal history.

The Remainder. Of the total 94 boys, 65 are included in the above groups. The remaining 29 boys (16 Reading and 13 Spelling Retardates) do not constitute a "group" in that they are not linked together on the Minimum

Spanning Tree. However, 21 cluster around 4 cases at the end of the MST opposite to the "genetic" group. The frequencies of most atypical responses conform to those found in all 94 boys, but some are considerably higher. On the Benton Test of Visual Retention, 52 per cent performed below the level expected for age and IQ. On the tests of finger localization, 44 per cent scored at the 5th percentile or below on one or both tests. The perinatal history was abnormal in 34 per cent of the boys.

Discussion

The fact that clusters did not emerge naturally does not support the existence of clearly defined types of dyslexia in this sample. One probable reason why no clusters were evident is that some features, for example, low scores on sound blending, Digit Span and Coding and lack of hand-eye-foot concordance, occur so frequently that they are unlikely to differentiate one group from another. Another reason may be that this highly selected sample was too homogeneous to include sub-groups.

Together both groups of dyslexics present a continuum of degrees of reading backwardness. Severely or moderately dyslexic boys showed no tendency to cluster separately but are evenly distributed throughout the Minimum Spanning Tree. If the severely retarded were characterized by features quite different from the moderately retarded, it could be expected that these differing features might provide some basis for clusters. That this did not occur strengthens the conclusion that their disorders are essentially of a similar nature. If there should be any heterogeneity, it would not appear to be based on the degree of reading retardation.

No explanation is offered for the unusual and unexpected responses on the examination of tendon reflexes, knee to ankle movement and eye movements. Of the three, the knee to ankle test is the only one which carries neurological significance, being used as a test for gross incoordination and ataxia. The minor degree of abnormal movement recorded here as a positive test would not usually be given such an interpretation. It was therefore surprising that minor abnormalities on the knee to ankle and the eye movement tests were found to occur statistically more frequently among the dyslexic boys. Their association with perinatal complications in Group 3 raises the possibility that they are signs of neurological dysfunction. The composition of the continuum evident from the MST suggests that in a few cases a dyslexia of genetic origin can be distinguished from one possibly acquired and associated with minor neurological dysfunction. But the fact that these minimal signs, birth hazards and positive family histories are found in conjunction with each other throughout the continuum suggests that specific dyslexia is seldom due to a single factor, as theories of its genetic or exogenous origin have so commonly upheld.

The patterns of impairment found in our four artificially created groups show both differences and similarities. Group 2 conforms most closely to previous descriptions of specific dyslexia of genetic origin. The term "Specific Language Disability," used in the past by the Orton Society, would seem to be a most appropriate label. The characteristics of this group bear a strong resemblance to that group of children described by Ingram (1964) as typified by speech-sound difficulties and to the auditory dyslexic described by Johnson and Myklebust (1967).

In Group 3, the perinatal histories and the presence of multiple minor neurological signs strongly suggest that the specific reading retardation is associated with some form of cerebral insult. The pattern of disabilities relates to the same visuo-spatial and visual retention deficits that are said to be characteristic of brain-injured children (Strauss and Kephart, 1955; Francis-Williams, 1970). Speech disorders are also found and each boy shows indeterminate hand or foot preference.

Group 4 can be regarded as a second "genetic" group. Although the boys are few in number, they are in many respects unlike those in Group 2. Speech and language, apart from reading and spelling, are relatively unaffected. Laterality is less fully established. Minor neurological signs, isolated and not multiple as in Group 3, are more common. On the Bristol Social Adjustment Guide scores suggestive of instability are more common in this group than any other. There is no hint from the history or findings suggestive of an acquired neurological dysfunction.

Group 1 is the only group of reasonable size to be identified by severing the MST at a distance threshold of 18·5. Within the limits of the information obtained in this study, no clue is provided as to the aetiology of the learning difficulty. Family histories of reading or spelling difficulties and perinatal abnormality are conspicuous by their almost complete absence. No unusually high frequency of response or pattern of disability is found to distinguish this group from others. Yet in all but 4 boys there is evidence of developmental delay or disorder.

Although some patterns of disability, immaturity or atypical response occur with greater frequency in some groups than in others, none is confined to any one group. The response made by a child to any task will be influenced and determined by a number of conditions and, conversely, a number of conditions may give rise to a single type of response. For example, an articulatory defect may simply reflect the standard of speech in the environment. It may also be due to faulty hearing or to an inability to co-ordinate the movements required to produce the sound and these in turn may be due to a developmental delay or to neurological impairment. A combination of conditions may be at work. The inco-ordination shown by a number of boys in each of the four groups may reflect a developmental delay in most but may be associated with neurological impairment in some. Similarly, the speech and language disorders would appear to have a genetic basis in Group 2 but this is not so likely in the case of the boys in Group 3. Zangwill's (1960) suggestion, that poorly developed laterality and reading retardation occurring together may be the effects of a cerebral lesion, may explain, in the absence of familial left-handedness, the high incidence of ambilaterality among the boys in Group 3, whereas in Group 4 the atypical laterality patterns are more likely to be genetically determined. In many boys only a multiple aetiology could explain their disorders. In the individual boys in this sample, it is impossible on clinical or psychological grounds to distinguish between a dyslexia of presumptive genetic origin, one acquired as a result of brain damage and one for which no clear cause can be ascertained.

Not only are no disabilities confined to any one group but some occur frequently in all, particularly low scores on sound blending, Digit Span and Coding. The classification of the WISC subtests into three categories, Verbal

Conceptualizing Ability, Spatial Ability and Sequencing Ability revealed that in all four groups, Sequencing Ability is considerably poorer than either Verbal or Spatial Abilities. This evidence of a sequencing disability, which may underlie or in some way cause the reading and spelling retardation, is supported by Doehring's (1968) conclusion that a disturbance of sequential organization, both verbal and visual, lies at the root of specific reading difficulties. The processes involved in carrying out tasks like sound blending and the repetition of a sequence of digits are complex and a defect in executing the composite act could be due to a defect in one or more of the necessary component skills.

It is perhaps significant that the only group, Group 1, to comprise boys between whom the similarity coefficients were high, should form the "core" of the Minimum Spanning Tree. The disorders of the boys in this group are varied and isolated and would seem to reflect differential rates of maturation rather than true abnormality. Different aspects of brain function mature at different rates and such differential growth of brain function may be much more pronounced in some children than in others and be responsible for widely varying rates in the acquisition of different types of skill, some lagging far behind others. A marked unevenness in the rate at which particular skills are acquired will then become apparent. The developmental "lag" may be specific to sensori-motor, verbal or visual skills, but when it affects skills intimately involved in learning to read, write and to spell, specific dyslexia and dysgraphia are likely to follow. Since reading, writing and spelling involve so many skills, the clinical picture is likely to vary from child to child. The delay in neurological and functional development may be the result of normal genetic variants. Children constitutionally so predisposed may be more liable to stress or to other special circumstances affecting different types of learning. Birth hazards, which leave most babies unscathed, may exacerbate congenital weaknesses and cause additional handicaps which lead to a consequent severe learning difficulty.

Some learning delay or defect other than the reading and spelling difficulty was found in all but a few boys. In the term "specific dyslexia" the adjective "specific" is valid only in so far as it describes the appreciable discrepancy between general intellectual potential and the standards attained in reading and spelling.

The absence of clearly defined sub-groups and the indications of a multiple rather than a unitary causation do not support the view that aetiologically or clinically separate forms of dyslexia can be distinguished. Unfortunately, the diagnosis of "specific dyslexia" is limited by many workers to a dyslexia of generic origin. It would seem more appropriate to use "specific dyslexia" to describe those learning disorders in which the *major* defect lies in learning to read, write and spell, the disability usually being accompanied by other developmental defects, for example, in speech, perceptual, constructional and arithmetic skills. The basis of the learning difficulty may be inherited, acquired as the result of early brain damage, symptomatic of a minimal neurological dysfunction or a combination of these. It is important to recognize that the learning failure is not primarily the result of deficient educational opportunity or of severe emotional disturbance.

12

Summary, Conclusions and Implications

This investigation attempts to clarify some issues relating to the existence, nature and causes of specific dyslexia. Many affirm that a constitutional disorder selectively affecting the ability to learn to read and to spell, exists, but many deny it. The denial seems to be based partly on some confusion about what is implied by the term "specific dyslexia" and partly on the difficulty of identifying the disorder as a single syndrome. Another reason for the denial may be that in any group of children who are finding difficulty in learning to read, it is both easy and correct to blame low intelligence, environmental conditions, unsuitable conventional instruction and primary emotional disturbance for the failure. Our concern in this study is the relatively small group for whom these do not provide the explanation.

These issues are of more than theoretical importance. To be unable to read or write has a crippling effect on the education, emotional well-being and future prospects of children. If there be children the nature of whose disorder demands facilities for examination and treatment not normally provided, their recognition has the practical importance that appropriate help and support cannot be given without it. During the years of this investigation, the Chronically Sick and Disabled Persons Bill has been enacted, which includes a clause relating to the provision of facilities for the assessment and treatment of dyslexic children. This alone gives added urgency to the need for recognition.

The objectives of this investigation were to identify those features by which boys who conformed to an accepted definition of specific dyslexia might be recognized. In view of the contention that the disorder with which we are concerned is merely one which is found at the lowest end of a continuum of reading skill, the experiment was designed to include a group whose reading difficulty could not be so described. A further objective was to discover evidence which might support or refute hypotheses as to the causes of the disability. Lastly, in view of suggestions made in recent years that there may be sub-groups or types of dyslexia characterized by different patterns of disability, an attempt is made by cluster analysis to distinguish such patterns and to relate them to the various possible aetiological factors.

The subjects are 98 dyslexic boys, selected from 271 boys examined at the Word Blind Centre for Dyslexic Children between January 1967 and

March 1969. They ranged in age from 8 years to 12 years 11 months and met the following criteria: Full Scale IQ on the Wechsler Intelligence Scale for Children (WISC) not less than 90, the Verbal IQ in no case less than 85; normal on physical and classical neurological examination; emotionally stable, and without major absence from school, especially during the first two years and no more than three changes of school. The 98 dyslexics were divided into two groups, one of 56 boys, designated Reading Retardates, retarded by 2 years or more in reading ability, the other of 42 boys, Spelling Retardates, retarded by 2 or more years in spelling and with a reading quotient derived from IQ and age of less than 80 but in no case is the reading retardation as severe as that in any Reading Retardate. Each of the two dyslexic groups was matched for age and type of school with a similar number of boys unselected for reading ability or for IQ except for the lower limits applied to the dyslexics. Since the dyslexics were predominantly middle-class, the controls were drawn from schools in these middle-class areas of London.

All boys were given a full general medical and neurological examination. Obstetric reports for most boys born in hospital were obtained. The psychological examination included the administration of the WISC, tests of reading and of spelling, of auditory discrimination, articulation, sound blending, right/left discrimination, motor proficiency, visual retention, finger localization and tests of hand, eye and foot preference. Information obtained from the parents included details of developmental history, illness, behavioural problems, mother/child separations and the presence of left-handedness and of difficulties in reading, spelling and speech in the child's immediate family. Details of school attendance, parental interest, and an estimate of intelligence on a five-point scale were obtained from schools where the Bristol Social Adjustment Guide (The Child in School) was completed.

The summary of the results is divided into three sections. The first reports findings which result from a comparison of each dyslexic group and its control group, two comparisons being made for each variable. When a difference has been found between only one dyslexic group and its control, this is stated. Otherwise both groups of dyslexics are referred to as "dyslexics" and both groups of controls as "controls." The second section indicates the areas of similarity and difference between the two dyslexic groups, and the third section reports the results of a cluster analysis.

Summary: Section 1

Home and family. The majority of both dyslexics and controls come from the two upper socio-economic classes. Only a small minority of mothers had worked or were working either full or part time and mother/child separations during the first four years for reasons of work or otherwise were no more frequent among the dyslexics than among the controls. Fewer Reading Retardates were eldest children (the difference just fails to reach the 5 per cent level of significance). Very few parents of boys in all groups were said by the school to be uninterested or only slightly interested in their sons' progress or behaviour at school. A family history of reading difficulty was reported more frequently among the dyslexics than among the controls, the level of significance being higher in the case of the Spelling Retardates. In this clinic sample, the percentages of dyslexic and of control boys with a positive family history, 36·7 per cent and 11·5 per cent respectively, are remarkably similar to the percentages found in a total population sample, among children with a specific reading retardation and a control group, 33·7 per cent and 9·2 per cent respectively (Rutter, Tizard and Whitmore 1970). No significant differences were found with regard to familial speech difficulties or left-handedness, although both are more frequently reported among the dyslexics.

School. The control boys were reading and spelling, on average, in advance of chronological age. By comparison with boys of the same age, in the same type of school and from a similar background, the retardation of the dyslexic boys is more marked than the discrepancy between chronological and reading or spelling ages indicates. No dyslexic boy attended a grammar school. Seven were at a secondary modern school and 4 of these were of grammar school intellectual calibre. Extra help with reading had been given to 68 dyslexics, 70·8 per cent, but only 15 boys had received help in a recognized remedial situation, either in a remedial class or from a visiting remedial teacher.

Behaviour. Behavioural problems at home were neither more numerous nor more frequent among dyslexics than among controls. Boys whose report from school had suggested maladjustment were excluded from this sample. Notwithstanding this, school reports give the impression that behaviour problems are more common at school among the Reading Retardates.

Neurological aspects. A greater number of Reading Retardates did not walk unaided until the age of 15 months or later. Early clumsiness was noted more frequently by parents of dyslexic boys than by parents of the control boys. Dyslexics were later in using sentences than controls and were also later in acquiring intelligible speech. Early articulatory defects were reported for a greater number of dyslexics than controls but early language difficulties were significantly more common only among the Reading Retardates. On the test of motor proficiency, only the Reading Retardates gave a significantly poorer performance. But the Spelling Retardates included a greater number of boys who showed poor control on the knee to ankle movement test and a nystagmoid eye movement. No differences were found on the tests of finger localization. A difficulty in differentiating between right and left occurred more commonly only among the Reading Retardates. This group includes more left-handed writers but it is indeterminate hand dominance rather than strong left-handedness which is the more striking feature and which distinguishes the Reading Retardates not only from their controls but also from all boys, excluding those in this sample, who were examined at the Centre while this sample was being collected. The Spelling Retardates include fewer consistently right-eyed boys and a greater number who were inconsistent in eye preference. A higher incidence of cross-laterality distinguishes the Spelling Retardates both from their controls and from other Centre cases. This also applies to the low frequency with which unilateral concordance between hand, eye and foot was found.

Perinatal history. On the physician's assessment of perinatal conditions, an abnormal history was no more frequent among dyslexics than among controls. A greater number of mothers of dyslexic boys reported illnesses during pregnancy, but these included illnesses which were unlikely to affect the developing foetus. Information on the presence or absence of an Rh negative factor was obtained in only 83 of all cases. An Rh– factor appeared to be more frequent in the mothers of dyslexic boys but differences are not statistically significant. Four boys were twins, all dyslexic. No differences were found between mean birth weights, but six boys were premature by birth weight, all dyslexics. Neonatal problems were no more frequent among dyslexic boys than among control boys.

Wechsler Intelligence Scale for Children. Dyslexics obtained significantly lower scores than controls on Information, Arithmetic, Digit Span and Coding. The Reading Retardates were in addition poorer on Vocabulary, Similarities and Block Design. Verbal IQ is lower than Performance IQ more frequently only among the Reading Retardates. Differences of 20 points or more between Verbal and Performance IQ were not found to be more common among the dyslexics. Where such differences were found they revealed a higher Verbal IQ as often as a higher Performance IQ. No differences of IQ were found between the Spelling Retardates and their controls but all IQs were lower in the case of the Reading Retardates.

Articulation. On examination, dyslexics made more errors than controls on the test of articulation. Moderately or severely defective articulation was found only among dyslexics.

Sound blending. Dyslexics made more errors on a task requiring them to blend sounds, the difficulty being more marked among the Reading Retardates.

Auditory Discrimination. No differences were found between dyslexics and controls.

Visual Retention. In reproducing designs from memory, the Reading Retardates made more errors and produced fewer correct designs than their controls. But when age and IQ are taken into account, no difference is found.

Summary: Section 2

Similarities between Reading and Spelling Retardates

In both groups delays in speech development, early articulatory difficulties and early clumsiness are more frequently reported. On examination, both groups gave evidence of some inco-ordination, of atypical patterns of laterality and of low scores on the tests of articulation and of sound blending. Scores on the WISC subtests of Information, Arithmetic, Digit Span and Coding were low. No differences were found between the dyslexic groups on the subtests of Comprehension, Similarities, Digit Span, Picture Completion, Picture Arrangement, Object Assembly or Coding nor were differences between Verbal and Performance IQ greater in one group than in the other. On the test of visual retention, no difference was found with respect to the number of designs correctly reproduced or the number of errors made.

Differences between Reading and Spelling Retardates

In addition to the delays and deficits found in both groups of dyslexic boys, only the Reading Retardates included a significantly greater number who had shown early language difficulties; their mean score on the WISC Vocabulary subtest was lower than that of the Spelling Retardates and the Verbal IQ more frequently lower than Performance IQ. The mean scores of the Reading Retardates are lower than those of the Spelling Retardates on Information, Arithmetic and Block Design. The mean total score on the test of right/left discrimination is lower than that of the Spelling Retardates.

Summary: Section 3

A cluster analysis was carried out to discover whether sub-groups or types of dyslexia could be identified. No clear clusters or groups emerged to support the existence of clearly definable sub-groups. Instead there appeared to be a continuum in one half of which there was a predominance of boys with a family history of reading or spelling difficulty while in the other half were found the majority of a smaller number of boys in whom there was evidence suggestive of neurological dysfunction but a negative family history. Four groups were artifically but legitimately created on the hypothesis that a genetically determined dyslexia could be distinguished from one associated with a minor neurological condition. Tests of the statistical significance of the differences in the frequency of the variables submitted to the cluster analysis were not made. Some striking differences between the groups suggest that there may be more than one type of genetic dyslexia, one characterized by speech and language delays and disorders, and another by atypical patterns of laterality. In one small group, a history of perinatal abnormality and findings suggestive of neurological dysfunction appear to be associated with a specific difficulty in reproducing visual patterns from memory and, to a lesser degree, speech disorder. One group, which seemed to lie at the centre of the continuum, is remarkable for the almost complete absence of positive family histories or perinatal conditions that might have adversely affected the central nervous system. Nevertheless, all but 4 boys in this group showed some delay or deficit although in differing areas of function. No disability was restricted to any one group. Common to all groups were a high frequency of difficulty in blending a sequence of sounds into a whole word and low scores on Digit Span and Coding, all involving a serial ordering process. In most boys, complex rather than single aetiological factors appear to be operative and it would seem that specific dyslexia seldom occurs in so isolated a form as hypotheses relating to genetic or acquired dyslexia might suggest.

Conclusions

This is a study of 98 boys retarded in reading and spelling. They are of at least average intelligence, normal on physical and classical neurological examination, emotionally stable, with continuous schooling and pre-dominantly from upper and middle class.

The following conclusions are drawn:

The results of this investigation support the concept that some reading and spelling disorders are constitutionally determined.

The evidence from this study does not support the existence of clearly defined sub-types of dyslexia.

Patterns of disability vary but there is evidence to suggest that a sequencing disability may underlie the reading and spelling retardation.

The importance in the aetiology of specific dyslexia of developmental neurological anomalies, some genetic, some acquired, is demonstrated.

Only a multiple aetiology would account for the observations in many boys. Varying aetiological factors seem to be associated with different patterns of disability, but these patterns are insufficiently distinct to allow a clear-cut identification of sub-types.

Greater similarities than differences are found between boys who exhibit a severe dyslexia and those showing a lesser reading difficulty but whose spelling remains a handicap, suggesting that their disorders are of an essentially similar nature.

Family histories of reading and of spelling difficulty are significantly commoner in these dyslexic boys than in their controls.

There is no greater frequency of mother/child separations, behaviour problems, early illness, birth hazards nor difference in birth weight, birth or family order when the dyslexics are compared with controls.

Although the majority of these dyslexic boys had been given much assistance, only 15 had received *remedial* tuition. All were still experiencing considerable difficulty, indicating that the help given was inadequate.

Implications and Recommendations

One of the main reasons for the importance of accepting the concept of a specific dyslexia is that only the awareness of *all* likely reasons for a child's failure to learn to read ensures that the necessary steps are taken to identify those factors operative in the individual child. An awareness that emotional disturbance can block learning, or that some inadequacy in environmental conditions can lie at the root of the problem, leads to a full inquiry into these conditions. The recognition that a reading disorder may result from constitutional developmental anomalies should lead to those investigations most likely to reveal evidence of their presence. In this study such evidence was found only by a full medical and psychological examination. Facilities for such investigations do exist in most parts of the country. But, to quote from the last report of the Chief Medical Officer of the Department of Education and Science on the Health of the School Child (1969): "The school health and the school psychological services face a big problem in the investigation of these children and the medical role is crucial. Some local education authorities arrange for the examination of these children during the course of the routine work of school doctors and educational psychologists; others, such as Nottingham, provide a special dyslexia clinic. What is certain is that the few national clinics, such as the Word Blind Centre, set up by the Invalid Children's Aid Association in London, cannot alone meet the need."

The specific and isolated deficits characteristic of specific dyslexia are unlikely to be elicited on a routine medical examination or on a psychological examination which includes only an intelligence test and a test of reading. A full neurological examination and the examination of a wide range of psychological functions are necessary. The setting up of special clinics with a multi-disciplinary staff each, if necessary, covering a wide area would be one way of providing the necessary facilities for investigation.

The recognition of these developmental neurological disorders is an essential first step before plans can be made both for appropriate investigations and appropriate remedies.

Children who exhibit unusual patterns of learning disability require unusual and specialized methods of teaching. There are far too few trained remedial teachers to give such necessary tuition. The class teacher does her best, but when there is a specific impairment in the pupil's capacity to learn to read she is likely to meet with limited sucess. The difficulties of dyslexic children have to be understood. Learning abilities and disabilities vary from child to child. Knowledge of these and of how these disabilities impede learning is needed, if a teacher is to understand why one method is suited to one child but not to another. Familiarity with a wide range of methods, programmes and tools enables her to select those most likely to be effective in each child's case. Dyslexic children need such specialized teaching. Only if their disorder is recognized are they likely to receive it. A mistaken diagnosis or failure of recognition results in inappropriate treatment or none at all.

When a severe spelling difficulty is the major problem a child is disabled in expressing on paper what he can state orally. To the child this is no minor handicap. At present remedial services are rarely available to these children and should be extended to include them.

Remedial services cannot be extended without increasing the number of trained remedial teachers. There is a great need for many more courses for training teachers to deal with specific learning disabilities. Lectures, discussions, and visits to schools, both normal and special, will continue to play an important part in such courses. But first-hand experience of the difficulties to be encountered and of how to overcome them is the most effective way of learning about them. There should be much greater provision of opportunity for remedial teachers in training to work with children over a period of time long enough to gain an understanding of the diversity of the problems they will meet.

Many questions remain to be answered. No conclusions can be drawn from this study about the incidence of specific dyslexia. The size of the problem may well vary from area to area and, if so, each Authority would have to determine the incidence within its own area in planning to provide adequate facilities for assessment and treatment.

A difficulty in blending sounds was commonly found among the dyslexics. Blending sounds involves the perception, retention, recall and rapid reproduction in a precise order of a sequence of sounds. We have observed at the Centre that while some children improve in their ability to deal with sound sequences others do not, and these make little progress in learning to read. If we knew clearly the nature of the processes involved and how the processing of sequences might be facilitated, teaching techniques could be improved. Prospective instead of retrospective knowledge about the likelihood of improvement would be helpful in planning remedial programmes.

Many functions involved in learning to read have not been explored. Learning to read and to spell depend, in the last analysis, upon the ability of a child to form automatic and permanent associations between what he hears, says, sees and writes, and failure lies in an inability to make such lasting associations. If more were understood about the mechanisms involved and under what conditions *permanent* associations can be formed, new teaching methods could be devised.

In individual children different patterns of ability and disability are found. At the Word Blind Centre, the principle of working predominantly through the more strongly developed areas has had considerable, but not invariable, success but the effectiveness of this approach should be tested by controlled observation.

The need to identify at an early age the reason why a child is failing to learn to read is paramount. Failure of recognition leads to avoidable misery, anxiety, frustration and depression. How soon can developmental dyslexia be identified? Is it necessary to wait until pronouncement can be made with certainty? The investigations of de Hirsch, Jansky and Langford (1969) and McLeod (1969) indicate that it is possible to forecast, when children first go to school, those likely to find reading difficult. Jessie Francis-Williams's (1970) study of pre-school children suggests that children with specific learning difficulties can be picked out before they go to school. During the first year at school, teachers and school medical officers together could carry out effective screening. This would require the construction of a short battery of tests which teachers can be trained to give. The school medical examination could routinely include taking a history of speech and motor development and an evaluation of a child's present articulation, use of language and of his motor co-ordination, all significantly associated with specific dyslexia. Children who show a marked unevenness in their development could then be selected for fuller investigation. Screening, carried out at the beginning of schooling, would also provide data on incidence on which plans for future needs could be based. Early screening would also have an effect on the management of children. A teacher aware that a child shows unevenness of development and aware of the specific areas which are "out of step" would be in a better position to give the understanding and support so essential to emotional well-being. She could also ensure that the child is given the kind of help *he* needs, that his disabilities do not prevent the realization of his abilities. Preventive and supportive steps taken early are immeasurably more humane and fruitful than attempts to remedy a problem which becomes increasingly complex as the child grows older. Our concern is not only the reading disability but the total welfare of the child.

Appendix 1: Tables

Table 1

Parental Age at Birth of Child (comprising only the cases in which both parents' ages are known), in each Socio-economic Class

	Reading Retardates			Control 1			Spelling Retardates			Control 2		
	No.	Mean	SD	No.	Mean	SD	No.	Mean	SD	No.	Mean	SD
SE Class 1												
Mother	14	29·4	2·23	14	29·7	4·82	13	29·6	5·82	12	32·4	6·61
Father	14	33·4	4·64	14	33·0	6·81	13	34·8	7·71	12	33·9	6·13
SE Class 2												
Mother	23	29·1	4·80	28	30·4	5·62	25	29·1	4·38	14	31·1	5·68
Father	23	31·9	5·03	28	34·0	6·50	25	31·4	4·27	14	37·1	9·04
SE Class 3a												
Mother	5	29·6	2·87	4	24·0	4·95	1	30·0	–	4	28·7	3·77
Father	5	33·0	4·86	4	29·5	5·36	1	30·0	–	4	28·5	4·97
SE Class 3b												
Mother	10	32·1	5·52	7	28·4	4·98	2	31·0	5·00	5	31·4	3·56
Father	10	33·8	5·00	7	32·0	5·58	2	35·0	2·00	5	33·4	2·06
SE Class 4												
Mother	3	30·0	8·64	2	29·0	3·00	1	21·0	–	2	25·0	5·00
Father	3	36·7	11·15	2	31·0	4·00	1	24·0	–	2	28·0	5·00
SE Class 5												
Mother	0	–	–	0	–	–	0	–	–	1	21·0	–
Father	0	–	–	0	–	–	0	–	–	1	26·0	–
Total Classes												
Mother	55	29·8	4·74	55	29·5	5·48	42	29·2	5·00	38	30·7	5·98
Father	55	33·0	5·56	55	33·1	6·45	42	32·4	5·82	38	33·9	7·53

No statistically significant differences.

Mothers' age
Reading Retardates, Control 1 – Difference between means $p > 0.05$
Spelling Retardates, Control 2 – Difference between means $p > 0.05$

Fathers' age
Reading Retardates, Control 1 – Difference between means $p > 0.05$
Spelling Retardates, Control 2 – Difference between means $p > 0.05$

Difference between parents' ages
Reading Retardates, Control 1 – Difference between means $p > 0.05$
Spelling Retardates, Control 2 – Difference between means $p > 0.05$

Table 2
Boys Separated from Mother during the first 4 Years for Reasons
Other than Mother Working

	Reading Retardates	Control 1	Spelling Retardates	Control 2
Separation				
Yes	30	32	21	24
No	23	24	21	16
Unknown	3	0	0	2
Total number	56	56	42	42

Chi-square 1 d.f. $p > 0.05$.

Table 3
Teachers' Reports of Current School Attendance

	Reading Retardates	Control 1	Spelling Retardates	Control 2
Attendance				
Regular	44	39	37	30
Occasional absence	4	1	1	0
Frequent absence	0	1	0	0
Unknown	8	15	4	12
Total number	56	56	42	42

Table 4
The Type of Help given to 68 Dyslexics (43 Reading and 25 Spelling Retardates)

| | State School | | Private School | | |
	Reading Retardates	Spelling Retardates	Reading Retardates	Spelling Retardates	Total
Individual help from school teacher only	6	5	7	4	22
Special classes *only*	1	7	0	0	8
Special classes + *individual help**	0	0	2	1	3
Special classes + *remedial class*	1	0	0	0	1
Special classes + *CGC†*	2	0	0	1	3
Total	4	7	2	2	15
Special group *only*	4	2	2	1	9
Special group + *individual help*	2	0	2	0	4
Special group + *remedial class*	2	0	1	0	3
Special group + *remedial class + individual help*	1	0	0	0	1
Special group + *CGC*	2	0	1	0	3
Total	11	2	6	1	20
Peripatetic Remedial Teacher *only*	1	0	0	1	2
Peripatetic Remedial Teacher + *individual help*	1	0	1	0	2
Peripatetic Remedial Teacher + *remedial class*	1	0	0	0	1
Total	3	0	1	1	5
Remedial class *only*	3	0	0	0	3
Remedial class + *individual help*	1	0	0	0	1
Remedial class + *special class*	1	0	0	0	1
Remedial class + *special group*	2	0	1	0	3
Remedial class + *special group + individual help*	1	0	0	0	1
Remedial class + *Peripatetic Remedial Teacher + individual help*	1	0	0	0	1
Total	9	0	1	0	10
Child Guidance Clinic *only*	1	0	0	0	1
CGC + *individual help*	0	0	0	1	1
CGC + *special class*	2	0	0	1	3
CGC + *special group*	2	0	0	1	3
Total number	5	0	0	3	8
Total	38	14	17	11	80

*"Individual help" implies from school teacher, generally class teacher.
†CGC – Child Guidance Clinic.

Since so many boys received more than one type of help the sum total of this table does not correspond to the total number of boys who had been helped.

Table 5
Teachers' Estimate of Intelligence and WISC IQ Verbal (V) and
Performance (P) in Relation to Type of School and Knowledge of IQ on
Prior Testing 89 dyslexics and 80 Unselected Readers (Control)

Type of School	IQ known				IQ not known			
	Private		State		Private		State	
IQ	V	P	V	P	V	P	V	P
Rated Very Bright								
Dyslexic			120	110	137	125	116	98
Control					150	132	150	152
							149	115
					131	104	139	120
					121	110	137	128
							134	120
							131	138
							130	108
							126	127
							126	120
							120	131
							116	129
							116	115
Rated Bright								
Dyslexic	125	118	123	143	125	120	149	122
	124	121	123	128	124	117	126	124
	109	99	121	115	121	121	124	115
			113	113	110	94	123	128
					109	113	120	127
					106	103	116	136
					100	120	114	111
							109	108
							100	117
Control					155	127	134	125
					137	111	128	133
					135	131	128	118
					135	128	126	121
					134	138	126	121
					129	128	109	108
					128	111	108	103
					125	140	105	121
					125	122	105	117
					123	124		
					123	103		
					121	127		
					113	132		
Rated Average								
Dyslexic	138	127	109	111	129	127	128	113
	120	97	109	100	124	103	121	132
	118	125	105	117	121	136	119	114
	113	104	105	110	121	127	119	110
	108	120	103	125	118	121	116	107
	95	99	103	122	116	121	115	125
			100	106	106	118	114	115
			97	99	106	104	111	131
			92	104	101	106	111	110

| Type of School | IQ known | | | | IQ not known | | | |
| | Private | | State | | Private | | State | |
IQ	V	P	V	P	V	P	V	P
Rated Average (continued)								
Dyslexic					99	111	111	93
					95	114	110	96
					90	104	106	106
							104	110
							103	105
							101	97
							99	117
							99	108
							97	86
							95	101
							86	97
Control					147	118	126	118
					135	120	126	117
					133	121	119	120
					130	124	119	117
					121	115	119	104
					121	110	118	101
					121	101	115	124
					120	107	115	92
					119	121	114	124
					118	115	113	103
					114	113	110	115
					113	117	109	124
					110	90	106	121
					109	104	106	101
					108	114	106	101
							105	104
							104	93
							103	87
							100	117
							100	103
							96	93
							95	127**
Rated Below Average								
Dyslexic	104	106	109	103	115	114	120	128
	101	107	106	87	112	129	97	110
	96	97	100	89	105	96		
			91	93				
Control					119	108*	110	104
					113	115	101	101
							89	120**
Rated Limited								
Dyslexic			96	111	116	87	118	111
							89	99
Control							87	111

*Severe spelling difficulty.
**Reading and Spelling difficulty.

Table 6
Test of Motor Proficiency. Chronological Age Levels and Performance Commensurate or Not Commensurate with Age
Reading Retardates and Control 1

Age Level	8 and 9 yrs		10 yrs		11 and 12 yrs	
Group	Reading Retardates	Control 1	Reading Retardates	Control 1	Reading Retardates	Control 1
Commensurate	6	13	4	7	8	12
Not Commensurate	14	7	12	8	10	8
Total number	20	20	16	15	18	20

$p < 0.05$

Spelling Retardates and Control 2

Group	Spelling Retardates	Control 2	Spelling Retardates	Control 2	Spelling Retardates	Control 2
Commensurate	9	15	8	6	3	2
Not Commensurate	11	9	5	5	4	5
Total number	20	24	13	11	7	7

Table 7
Right/Left Discrimination

	Reading Retardates No.	M	Control 1 No.	M	Spelling Retardates No.	M	Control 2 No.	M
Own Body Eyes Open								
8 years	9	8·0	8	9·9	11	8·3	12	8·7
9 years	10	5·2	12	8·7	9	9·4	12	9·9
10 years	14	8·9	16	9·8	13	9·2	11	9·5
11 years	11	7·9	8	9·9	6	10·0	5	9·6
12 years	8	9·6	12	9·8	1	10·0	2	9·5
Total	52	7·9	56	9·6***	40	9·2	42	9·4
Own Body Eyes Open								
8 years	9	4·8	8	6·0	11	4·9	12	5·7
9 years	10	3·7	12	5·4	9	5·9	12	5·9
10 years	14	5·2	16	6·0	13	5·8	11	5·7
11 years	11	5·6	8	6·0	6	6·0	5	6·0
12 years	8	5·6	12	6·0	1	6·0	2	6·0
Total	52	5·0	56	5·9***	40	5·6	42	5·8
Other Person								
8 years	9	2·7	8	3·6	11	1·8	12	2·6
9 years	10	1·6	12	3·4	9	1·3	12	3·5
10 years	14	2·6	16	2·9	13	3·1	11	3·4
11 years	11	2·2	8	4·0	6	4·0	5	3·6
12 years	8	3·6	12	3·8	1	4·0	2	2·0
Total	52	2·5	56	3·5***	40	2·9	42	3·1
Total score	52	15·4	56	18·9***	40	17·7	42	18·3

***Difference between means significant at the 0·1% level.

Table 8
History of Illnesses

	Reading Retardates	Control 1	Spelling Retardates	Control 2
Mumps				
No	21	27	14	22
Yes (CR age)	17	1	14	1
Yes under 5 years	6	12	5	9
over 5 years	12	15	8	8
Total number	56	55	41	40
Chicken Pox				
No	9	9	7	11
Yes (CR age)	22	0	15	1
Yes under 5 years	8	24	6	13
over 5 years	13	23	8	15
Total number	52	56	36	40
Measles				
No	6	5	3	5
Yes	45	51	34	35
Total number	51	56	37	40
German Measles				
No	19	30	10	16
Yes	21	24	18	23
Total number	40	54	28	39
Poliomyelitis				
No	56	54	42	40
Yes under 5 years	0	2	0	0
Total number	56	56	42	40
Encephalitis				
No	56	55	42	40
Yes over 5 years	0	1	0	0
Total number	56	56	42	40
Rheumatic Fever				
No	55	56	42	40
Yes over 5 years	1	0	0	0
Total number	56	56	42	40
Jaundice				
No	50	55	39	38
Yes under 5 years	4	1	3	0
over 5 years	0	0	0	2
Total number	54	56	42	40
Convulsions/Fits				
No	52	55	36	40
Yes under 5 years	1	1	1	0
Total number	53	56	37	40

Chi-square 1 d.f. − each illness − $p > 0.05$.

Table 9
Incidence of Accidents (Head Injuries, Broken Bones, Severe Burns, Others), under and over Age 5

	Reading Retardates	Control 1	Spelling Retardates	Control 2
Accidents				
Under 5 years				
No	36	44	31	28
Yes	9	11	3	10
Total number	45	55	34	38
Accidents –				
Over 5 years				
No	30	40	29	28
Yes	11	12	5	7
Total number	41	52	34	35

Chi-square 1 d.f. $p > 0.05$ in each comparison.

Table 10
History of Asthma, Eczema and Headaches

	Reading Retardates	Control 1	Spelling Retardates	Control 2
Asthma				
No	51	51	40	40
Yes (CR age)	0	0	0	0
Yes less than 3 years	0	2	0	0
3 to 5 years	2	1	1	0
6 to 8 years	1	1	1	0
9 to 11 years	1	0	0	0
Total number	55	55	42	40
Eczema				
No	46	48	37	36
Yes (CR age)	1	2	0	0
Yes less than 3 years	4	4	4	3
3 to 5 years	2	2	1	1
6 to 8 years	1	0	0	0
9 to 11 years	1	0	0	0
Total number	55	56	42	40
Headaches				
No	36	50	33	28
Yes (CR age)	5	4	1	0
Yes 3 to 5 years	5	1	3	3
6 to 8 years	3	0	4	7
9 to 11 years	4	1	0	1
12+ years	0	0	0	1
Total number	53	56	41	40

Chi-square 1 d.f. $p > 0.05$ in each comparison.

Table 11
Place of Confinement

	Reading Retardates		Control 1		Spelling Retardates		Control 2	
Place of confinement								
Home	17	31%	12	25%	9	22%	7	17%
Hospital	35 ⎫	69%	36 ⎫	75%	31 ⎫	78%	29 ⎫	83%
Nursing Home	3 ⎭		8 ⎭		1 ⎭		4 ⎭	
Total number	55		56		41		40	

Chi-square 1 d.f. $p > 0.05$.

Appendix 2: Record Forms and Questionnaires

Confidential   FAMILY INFORMATION

Please complete this form where applicable and return it to:—
*The Secretary, WORD BLIND CENTRE, Invalid Children's Aid Association,
Coram's Fields, 93 Guilford Street, London WC1.*

You may have difficulty remembering some of the information requested in
this form. If such is the case write in Cannot Remember (or CR) but only as
a last resort, as even vague memories may help. The information you give will
also help other children as it will be used anonymously for research into Word
Blindness, as well as for the diagnosis of your own child.

	(1)	1
	(2)	(3)	(4)

Child's Full Name ....

Child's Date of Birth .... / .... / ...... Age ... yrs .... mths ...

Mother's Names .... Age .... yrs .....

Father's Names .... Age .... yrs .....

Father's Occupation ....

Position or Rank ....

Is Mother working now? Full time or part time ....

Name of Family Doctor ....

Doctor's Address ....

....

Children in the family. (Please list *all* the children in the family beginning
with the eldest, Indicate age, sex, and relationship to patient, e.g. sister,
half-brother, *adopted* etc. Write "patient" in relationship column against
the name of the child who is being referred to us.)

	Names of Children	Boy Girl	Date of Birth	Age	Relationship
Eldest	....	......	....	......	....
Next	....	......	....	......	....
Next	....	......	....	......	....
etc	....	......	....	......	....
	....	......	....	......	....
	....	......	....	......	....

128

DETAILS OF CHILD'S EDUCATION

For Office
Use Only

Name of Present School . . . .

Full Address of School . . . .

Name of Headmaster . . . .

Name of Class Teacher . . . .

Year and Type of Class. . . . .

Type of School: State . . . . Private . . . .   0, 1 (5) [ ]

Is it one sex only . . . . or mixed . . . . .   0, 1 (6) [ ]

If child is over 11 years, is he at Secondary Modern/
Technical/Comprehensive/Private/Grammar/Prep./
Other

No 1
Sec 2
Tech 3   (7)
Comp 4
Priv 5   [ ]
Gram 6
Prep 7
Other 8

DETAILS OF PREVIOUS SCHOOLS

Type of School
(Nursery,
Names of Schools   Junior, etc.)   Address   Class and Year

. . . .

. . . .   Code no
                                                                                        0, 1 . . . 9+
. . . .
                                                                                        (8)   [ ]
. . . .

. . . .

PREVIOUS TREATMENT OF CHILD'S DIFFICULTIES

(underline *all* cases which apply)

Has child had extra help *from* the School?   0, 1, 2, 3, 4
None/In special class/In special group/from visiting
remedial teacher/individual help from school teacher.   (9)   [ ]
Has child had help from *outside* School?   0, 1, 2, 3.
None/attended Child Guidance Clinic/attended
remedial class/from individual teacher.   (10)   [ ]
Has child been previously examined by a
psychologist?   No . . . . .   0 (11) [ ]
                                             Yes   1

(Please give details of any other treatment which the
child has had which is not covered above, e.g. speech
centres, visits to specialists, etc.)

. . . .

. . . .

. . . .

DEVELOPMENTAL MILESTONES

First tooth at . . . . months   (12, 13) ☐☐

Sitting up at . . . . months   (14, 15) ☐☐

Crawling at . . . . months   (16, 17) ☐☐

Walking with help at . . . . months   (18, 19) ☐☐

Walking without help at . . . . months   (20, 21) ☐☐

Have you noticed any signs of clumsiness?   (enter true
                                                                figures)
    No   0,
                                                              1, (22)   ☐
    Yes . . . .

SPEECH ACQUISITION

Mama/Dada spoken at. . . . . months   (23, 24) ☐☐

Additional 4 or 5 words at . . . . months   (25, 26) ☐☐

Full sentences of several words at . . months   (27, 28) ☐☐

Age at which pronunciation was clear to strangers   (29) ☐

    . . . . years   0, 1, . . .9+

Have parents noticed any articulatory defects?

    No   0,
                                                                     (30)☐
    Yes   1,

Have parents noticed any language difficulties?

    No   0,
                                                                     (31)☐
    Yes.   1,

Is English the only language spoken at home?

    No   0,
                                                                     (32)☐
    Yes   1,

Was child born in an English-speaking country? If not,
at what age did he come to live here?

Was born in an English-speaking country   0,
                                                                     (33)☐
Was not, but came here at . . . . years   1, 2, . . . 9+

0/1/2/3	For Office Use Only
Has the child had in the past or now got any of the following? Please *underline* in each case whichever applies. There is space below the list to write in further details if you so wish.	(Use code 0–3 from above)

Nervousness
Never/In the past/At present/In the past and at present   (34) ☐

Timidity
Never/In the past/At present/In the past and at present   (35) ☐

Fears of? (e.g. dark, etc)
Never/In the past/At present/In the past and at present   (36) ☐

Naughtiness
Never/In the past/At present/In the past and at present   (37) ☐

Jealousy or envy
Never/In the past/At present/In the past and at present   (38) ☐

Temper Tantrums
Never/In the past/At present/In the past and at present   (39) ☐

Silent Periods
Never/In the past/At present/In the past and at present   (40) ☐

Nightmares
Never/In the past/At present/In the past and at present   (41) ☐

Others? (e.g. Sleepwalking, etc)

No   0,

Yes . . . . .   (42) ☐

If yes, list . . . .   1, 2, . . . 9

0	1	2	3	4	5	6	For Office
Never	Yes	0–2	3–5	6–8	9–11	12 or over	Use Only

Has the child had in the past or got now any of the
following? Please underline *all ages* at which the
symptom occurred. If the age cannot be remembered
underline "Yes."

(i) occurring
(ii) recurring
(iii) again recurring.

Bed-wetting
Never/Yes (age unknown)/0–2/3/4/5/6/7/8/9/10/11/
12 or over/yrs

(43)   (44)   (45)

Soiling
Never/Yes/0–2/3/4/5/6/7/8/9/10/11/12 or over/yrs

(46)   (47)   (48)

Asthma
Never/Yes/0–2/3/4/5/6/7/8/9/10/11/12 or over/yrs

(49)   (50)   (51)

Eczema
Never/Yes/0–2/3/4/5/6/7/8/9/10/11/12 or over/yrs

(52)   (53)   (54)

Headaches
Never/Yes/0–2/3/4/5/6/7/8/9/10/11/12 or over/yrs

(55)   (56)   (57)

Others? (e.g. Vomiting, etc)

No . . . . . .

Yes . . . . .

If yes, list . . . .

(score 'O' if
(ii) or (iii)
do not apply

0,   (58)*

1, 2, ... 9

0	1	2	3	For Office Use Only

Has the child had any of the following illnesses? Please *underline* the appropriate answer.

Poliomyelitis
No/Yes-age not known/Pre-school (up to 5 yrs)/
During school age (Over 5 years) (59) ☐

Encephalitis
No/Yes-age not known/Under 5 years/Over 5 years (60) ☐

Rheumatic fever
No/Yes-age not known/Under 5 years/Over 5 years (61) ☐

Epilepsy
No/Yes-age not known/Under 5 years/Over 5 years (62) ☐

Convulsions or fits
No/Yes-age not known/Under 5 years/Over 5 years (63) ☐

Jaundice
No/Yes-age not known/Under 5 years/Over 5 years (64) ☐

Mumps
No/Yes-age not known/Under 5 years/Over 5 years (65) ☐

Chicken pox
No/Yes-age not known/Under 5 years/Over 5 years (66) ☐

Measles
No/Yes-age not known/Under 5 years/Over 5 years (67) ☐

German Measles
No/Yes-age not known/Under 5 years/Over 5 years (68) ☐

Bronchitis
No/Yes-age not known/Under 5 years/Over 5 years (69) ☐

Pneumonia
No/Yes-age not known/Under 5 years/Over 5 years (70) ☐

Fainting spells
No/Yes-age not known/Under 5 years/Over 5 years (71) ☐

No	0	/	1	/	2	/	3	/	4	/	5		For Office Use Only

Accidents

(a) Under 5 years: No . . . . . .   0.

Yes . . . . .   (72) ☐ *

If yes; Head injuries/broken bones/suffocation/severe   1, 2, 3, 4,
burns/other   5 . . . . .

(b) Over 5 years: No   0,

Yes . . . . .   (73) ☐ *

If yes; Head injuries/broken bones/suffocation/severe   1, 2, 3, 4,
burns/other   5 . . . . . .

Other Illnesses

No . . . . . .   Yes   0,

(74) ☐ *

If yes, list   1–9

Mother/Child Separation   Re-enter Sheet Code
Were mother and child ever separated from each other   (1) ☐ 2
for longer than one week during the *first four years*
of the child's life? Please note below *all* periods of   & Child
separation. (When stating who looked after the child,   ☐   ☐   ☐
choose from this classification: father/grandparents/   (2) (3) (4)
other relatives/nurse or nanny/close family friend/other.
If more than one applies, fill in both.) Use the second
column if there was more than one separation of one
kind.

(a) Did mother work at all during the first 4 years of
child's life?

No   0,   (75)
Yes . . . .   If yes, full-time . . . . . or part-time . . . . .   1, full   ☐
How old was the child then?   2, part
Less than 1/1 yr/2 yrs/3 yrs/4 yrs

Who looked after the child? . . . .   0–4 (76) ☐ *

Did the child stay: At home . . . . . . or elsewhere . . .   0–5 (77) ☐ *

(b) Mother in hospital?   1, 2 (78) ☐

No . . . .   Yes . . . .   (2nd occasion)   0,   (79) (80)

If yes, how long for?   1–3   ☐   ☐

How old was the child then?   . . . .   (5)
less than 1/1/2/3/4 years   0–4   ☐   ☐ (6)
(7) (8)

Who looked after the child?   0–5   ☐   ☐

Did the child stay: At home . . or elsewhere . . . . . .   1, 2   ☐   ☐
(9) (10)

Appendix 2 135

CODE: No –0; 1 wk–1; 1 wk to 1 month–2; more
than 1 month–3. Father–0; Grandparents–1;
relatives–2; nurse–3; friend–4; other–5.

For Office
Use Only

*For more than
one separation*

(c) Child in hospital?

    No . . . . . .   Yes . . . .   (11)   (12)

If yes, how long for? . . . .
How old was the child then?   (13)   (14)

Less than 1/1/2/3/4 yrs . . . . (15)   (16)

Who looked after the child?. . . . . , ,

Did the child stay: at home . . . . (17)   (18)

                elsewhere . . . .

(d) Holiday separation?   (19)   (20)

    No. . . . . . :   Yes . . . .

If yes, how long for? . . . . (21)   (22)
How old was the child then?

Less than 1/1/2/3/4 yrs . . . . (23)   (24)

Who looked after the child? . . . .

Did the child stay: at home . . . . . . , ... , (25)   (26)

               elsewhere   . . . . , ...

(e) Business separation?

    No . . . . . .   Yes . . . . (27)   (28)

If yes, how long for? . . . .
How old was the child then?   (29)   (30)

Less than 1/1/2/3/4 yrs . . . . , . . . (31)   (32)

Who looked after the child?. . . . .

Did the child stay: at home . . . . (33)   (34)

                elsewhere . . . .

(f) Other Separation

    No . . . . . .   Yes . . . .   (35)   (36)

How old was the child then?   (37)   (38)
Less than 1/1/2/3/4 yrs

Who looked after the child? . . . . (39)   (40)

Did the child stay: at home . . . . (41)   (42)

               elsewhere . . . . ,

Medical History of Child

Is hospital or medical record available?   No . . Yes . .

0, 1   (43) ☐

Pregnancy
Was the duration of pregnancy: normal full-term/
premature/overdue (39—41 wks)

n = 1
p= 2
o = 3, (44) ☐

If premature or overdue, by how many weeks? . . . . . .

o = No (45) ☐

Did you have any illnesses during pregnancy?   No . .

1, — 9+ wks

Yes . . .
If yes, write down their nature and how many weeks
pregnant you were at the time.

0, 1.

. . . .

. . . .

(46) ☐ *

. . . .

home = 1
Hosp = 2
n. home = 3

The Birth
Was the baby born at: home/hospital/nursing home?

(47) ☐

Name and address of Hospital or Clinic: . . . .

. . . .

(48)   (49)   (50)

Birth Weight. . . lbs . . ozs   (. . . ozs)

☐ ☐ ☐

Total length of labour in hours: . . . .

(51) ☐   ☐ (52)

Was delivery normal/caesarian/forceps-low-mid-high/
breech/P.O.P./other. Were there any other complications or unusual features about the birth?

(53) ☐

No/cord round neck/asphyxia/A.P.H./other . . . .

(54) ☐ *

Infancy
In the 4 weeks immediately following the birth did the
baby have any of the following?

0, 1 9

Jaundice	No	Yes	0, 1(55) ☐
Convulsions or fits	No	Yes	(56) ☐
High Temperatures	No	Yes	(57) ☐
Persistent crying	No	Yes	(58) ☐
Early Feeding Problems	No	Yes	(59) ☐
Other Illnesses	No	Yes	0, (60) ☐

If yes, list: . . . .

1, ... 9

Child's Difficulties and Symptoms:

Please describe below the disabilities from which your child suffers and for which you seek help. Include a brief history if possible. This section will be of great help to us.

Signed . . . .   Date . . . .

Relationship to Child . . . .
Please include with this a recent sample of the child's handwriting, e.g. a letter.

MEDICAL REPORT

Child's Full Name. . . . .   ( ) ( ) ( )
Child's Date of Birth. . /. . / . . . Age . . yrs. . mths. .   Child's number

Date of Interview . . . . Examiner . . . .   (5) sheet number

Child is Singleton/Twin -1st -2nd/Triplet -1st 2nd -3rd.   (50) ☐
Birth By Gestation   premature/full term/overdue
By Birth Weight   premature/not premature   (51) ☐

Pregnancy and Neonate   and   *Child's Illnesses*
check page 9   check pages 6 & 7
on Family Information Sheets

Perinatal
Presumed normal (home birth)   −1
Assumed normal (no way of checking)   −2
Normal (on basis of hospital report)   −3   (52) ☐

Physical Examination

Height . . . . ft . . . ins   = ... ins   (53, 54)   ☐☐

Weight . . . . st . . . lbs   = ... lbs   (55, 56, 57)☐☐☐

Vision Defects   −0 (no defect)
Defect (e.g. spectacles)/no defect/not known   1−9 defects
                                                                                    (58) ☐
If defect present list . . . .
Ears Normal/not normal
Heart Normal/not normal
Lungs Normal/not normal
Posture Normal/not normal
CNS Reflexes Normal/diminished/increased/   (59) ☐
exaggerated/with reinforcement
Spasticity Present/Absent

Physical condition   (60) ☐
Normal/Not normal
Knee to ankle test Normal/not normal   Pres −1   (61) ☐
Eye movement to Right Present/Absent   Abs −2   (62) ☐
Eye movement to Left Present/Absent   (63) ☐
                                                                          N − 1
Motor System   not N − 2   (64) ☐
Clumsiness Present/Absent
Incoordination Present/Absent   (65) ☐

Other Neurological Tests?   No − 0   Yes − 1   (66) ☐
If yes, Normal or Abnormal
                                                                          1, 2,
List. . . . .   3 . . . 9   (67) ☐

Audiometry?   No (0)   Yes (1)   (68) ☐

EEG?   No (0)   Yes (1)   (69) ☐

From Hospital Report Only
Mother RH−   No (0)   Yes (1)   (70) ☐
Baby Jaundice   No (0)   Yes (1)   (71) ☐

Other Complications   (72) ☐ *
List . . . .   (73) ☐ *
. . . .

```
┌─────────────────────────────────────────────────────────────┐
```

WORD BLIND CENTRE
Psychological Data

Sheet—(2)
child's
No. ( ) ( ) ( )
    (61) (62) (63)

Child's Name . . . .   ☐ ☐ ☐

Date of Birth . . . .   CA . . .⁼ . . . .   mths

Date of testing . . . Examiner . . . .   (64) ☐

(From Family Information Sheets)
Mother's Age (at birth of child) . . . . yrs
(65) (66) ☐   ☐

Father's Age (at birth of child) etc. . . . . yrs   (67) (68) ☐   ☐
Socio-Economic Status I/II/III/IV/V   (1, −5) (69) ☐
Is mother working now No—1/Full-time—2/Part-   (70) ☐
time—3
Is child: Natural—1/Adopted—2   (71) ☐

Parity
Within entire family 1st child (eldest)/2nd/3rd/   (72) ☐
4th/5th. . . . .   (72) ☐
In relation to mother her 1st child/2nd/3rd/4th/
5th. . . . .   (73) ☐

In Family
Number of brothers   0, 1, 2, 3, 4, 5, 6, 7, 8, 9+   (74) ☐
Number of sisters   0, 1, 2, 3, 4, 5, 6, 7, 8, 9+   (75) ☐
No. of half-brothers 0, 1, 2, 3, 4, 5, 6, 7, 8, 9+   (76) ☐
No. of half-sisters   0, 1, 2, 3, 4, 5, 6, 7, 8, 9+   (77) ☐
Foster brothers   0, 1, 2, 3, 4, 5, 6, 7, 8, 9+   (78) ☐
Foster sisters   0, 1, 2, 3, 4, 5, 6, 7, 8, 9+   (79) ☐

FAMILIAL HISTORY   sheet (1)   ☒
(From interview with parents). Have any members   No.
of the family had, or got now, any of the
characteristics listed below?   (2) (3) (4)
                                 ☐   ☐   ☐
(a) *Word Blindness or severe reading difficulties*

Father? No—0   Yes—1 . . . .(5)☐   Mother? No—0   Yes—1. . .(6)☐
Any brothers? No—0; 1,2,3,4,. .(7)☐   Any sisters? No—0; 1,2,3,4, . .(8)☐
½ brothers on F's side? 0,1,2,. .(9)☐   on M's side? 0,1,2,3,4, . . .(10)☐
½ sisters on F's side? 0,1,2,. . .(11)☐   on M's side? 0,1,2, 3, ...(12)☐

(b) *Late Reader*

Father? No—0 Yes—1 ..(13)☐	Mother? No—0 Yes—1 ..(14)☐
Any brothers? No—0; 1,2,3,4, (15)☐	.. sisters? No—0; 1,2,3,4, ...(16)☐
½ brothers on F's side? 0,1,2, (17)☐	.. on M's side? 0,1,2,3, ...(18)☐
½ sisters on F's side? 0,1,2,...(19)☐	.. on M's side? 0,1,2,3, ...(20)☐

(c) *Spelling Difficulties*

Father?? No—0 Yes—1... (21)☐	Mother? No—0 Yes—1..(22)☐
Any brothers? No—0; 1,2,3,4, (23)☐	Any sisters? No—0; 1,2,3,4, .(24)☐
½ brothers on F's side? 0,1,2,. (25)☐	on M's side? 0,1,2,3,4, ...(26)☐
½ sisters on F's side? 0,1,2, .. (27)☐	on M's side? 0,1,2,3,4, ...(28)☐

(d) *Left-Handedness*

Father? No—0 Yes—1 .. (29)☐	Mother? No—0 Yes—1 ..(30)☐
Any brothers? No—0; 1,2,3,4, (31)☐	Any sisters? No—0; 1,2,3,4, ..(32)☐
½ brothers on F's side? 0,1,2, (33)☐	on M's side? 0,1,2,3,4, ...(34)☐
½ sisters on F's side? 0,1,2, .. (35)☐	on M's side? 0,1,2,3,4, ...(36)☐

(e) *Mixed Laterality* (use the other hand a great deal e.g. sports, needlework, crafts)

Father? No—0 Yes—1 .. (37)☐	Mother? No—0 Yes—1 . (38)☐
Any brothers? No—0; 1,2,3,4, (39)☐	Any sisters? No—0; 1,2,3,4, .. (40)☐
½ brothers on F's side? 0,1,2, (41)☐	on M's side? 0,1,2,3,4, ... (42)☐
½ sisters on F's side? 0,1,2, .. (43)☐	on M's side? 0,1,2,3,4, ... (44)☐

(f) *Speech Difficulty*

Father? No—0 Yes—1 .. (45)☐	Mother? No—0 Yes—1 · (46)☐
Any brothers? No—0; 1,2,3,4, (47)☐	Any sisters? No—0; 1,2,3,4, · (48)☐
½ brothers on F's side? 0,1,2, (49)☐	on M's side? 0,1,2,3,4, ····· (50)☐
½ sisters on F's side? 0,1,2, .. (51)☐	on M's side? 0,1,2,3,4, ····· (52)☐

PSYCHOLOGICAL TESTS

1. *Laterality*   R−1
Preferred Hand.................,..... writing........   L−2   (53)□
Simultaneous Writing (General Handedness)
Strong R / R with L tendencies/Ambi/L with
R tendencies/Strong L.
   (0)   (1)   (2)   (3)   (4)   (54)□

Eyedness: Cards Asher's Test:.....................   R−1
                                                             L−2
            Kaleidoscope: .... V-scope: ......   A−3   (55)□
                                                             R−1
Footedness: Kicking:......... Hopping: ....   L−2   (56)□
Cross-lateral: Hand (writing)/Eye: A−3
No−0 R/L −1 L/R −2 R/A −3 L/A −4   (57)□
Dominance: Hand/Foot:
No−0 R/L −1 L/R −2 R/A −3 L/A −4   (58)□
Dominance: Hand/Eye/Foot: RH.RE.RF./LH.LE.LF./
Mixed   (1)   (2)   (59)□
(3)

2. *Wepman's Auditory Discrimination Test. Form A*   (60) (61)
                                                             □   □
Number of errors: .... ,........, ,...............
Normal = 0; Outside normal by 1, 2, 3, 4, 5, 6, 7, 8, 9+
points   (62)   □
Errors Present: v-th/f-th/m-n/a-e/k-p/b-g/b-d/d-g/s-f/   *
  (circle)   1   2   3   4   5   6   7   8   9   (63)   □
        th-sh/s-th/t-p/t-k/or-ur/e-i/oa-aw/s-sh/.   *
        1   2   3   4   5   6   7   8   (64)   □

3. *Benton's Right/Left Discrimination Test*   (65) (66)
Total Score:...............................   □   □
Sub-scores: Own body eyes open:.................   (67, 68)□ □
            Own body eyes closed:................   (69) □
            Picture: Other Person: ....   (70) □

4. *Sound Blending*   (71) (72)
Score:....................................   □   □

5. *Renfrew Articulation Attainment Test:*   (73) (74) (75)
Score:....................................   □   □   □
Articulatory defects in general conversation; No−0 Yes−1   (76) □

                                                             Sheet−(1)   ☑4
                                                             Child: □ □ □
                                                               (2) (3) (4)

6. *Schonell GWRT*   (77)   (78)   (79)
RA . . . . = ... months   ☐   ☐   ☐

7. *Schonell GWST*   (80)   (5)   (6)
SA . . . . = ... months   ☐   ☐   ☐
(a) Letter Reversals   None (0); 1 only (1); 2 or 3   (7)   ☐
    (from sentence)   (2); 4+ (3).
(b) Letter Transpositions No (0); 1 only (1); 2 or 3   (8)   ☐
                        (2); 4+ (3).
(c) Bizarre Spelling   No (0); 1 only (1); 2 or 3   (9)   ☐
    (jumble of letters) (2); 4+ (3).

8. *Neale Analysis of Reading Ability*   (10)   (11)   (12)
Rate . . . . = ... months   ☐   ☐   ☐
Accuracy . . . . = ... months (13,14,15) ☐   ☐   ☐
Comprehension . . . . = ... months (16,17,18) ☐   ☐   ☐
CA − RA (Acc) . . . . = ... months (19,20) ☐   ☐
CA − SA (Sch) . . . . = ... months (21, 22) ☐   ☐
RA − SA = · · · · · · · · · · · years (RA > by 4, 3, 2, 1 yr equal
                                 code----(0)(1)(2)(3)(4)   (23)
                                 RA less by 1, 2, 3, 4 yrs)   ☐
                                 (5)(6)(7)(8)
                                                             (24)   (25)   (26)
MA . . . . = ... months ☐   ☐   ☐
RQ . . . .(27,28,29) ☐   ☐   ☐
SQ . . . .(30,31,32) ☐   ☐   ☐

9. *WISC Full Scale IQ:* . . . . (33)(34)(35) ☐☐☐
                   (36)   (37)   (38)   (39)   (40)   (41)
Verbal IQ . . . . ☐   ☐   ☐ Performance IQ . . . ☐   ☐   ☐
Information . . . . . (42,43) ☐ ☐ Picture Completion (52,53)☐   ☐
Comprehension . . (44,45) ☐   ☐ Picture
Arithmetic . . . . . . (46,47) ☐ ☐ Arrangement . . . . (54,55)☐ ☐
Similarities . . . . . (48,49) ☐ ☐ Block Design . . . . (56,57)☐ ☐
Vocabulary . . . . . . (50,51) ☐ ☐ Object Assembly . (58,59) ☐ ☐
(Digit Span . . . . . . (62,63) ☐ ☐ Coding . . . . (60,61) ☐ ☐
Other IQ Test . . . . Date . . . .
Name and Details of Tester . . . .
. . . .

10. *Stott Test of Motor Proficiency* (in years)

Balance .... ☐ ☐(64,65)   *or Oseretsky*
Upper limb co-ordination ... ☐ ☐(66,67)   Balance ....(76,77) ☐ ☐
Whole body .... ☐ ☐(68,69)   Hand/Arm..... .(78,79) ☐ ☐
Manual dexterity .... ☐ ☐(70,71)   Speeded....... .(80,5) ☐ ☐
Simultaneous movement ... ☐ ☐(72,73)

(1)
Sheet ⑤

CA ....years   (74,75) ☐ ☐   Child's No
General Impairment Score .... (6) (7) ☐ ☐   (2) (3) (4)
                                                         ☐ ☐ ☐

11. *Synkinesis*

                    Flexion   Extension
In Part I: Absent/Mild or Marked/Mild or Marked/Present (unqualified) (8) ☐
            0   1   2   3   4   5
In Part II: Absent/Mild or Marked/Mild or Marked/Present   (9) ☐
            0   1   2   3   4   5
In Part III: Absent/Mild or Marked/Mild or Marked/Present   (10) ☐
            0   1   2   3   4   5

12. *Benton's Visual Retention Test. Form C. Administration A*
Number of designs correct ....(11,12) ☐ ☐
Within normal limits Normal/2 pts below/3 points/4 or more below   (13) ☐
                          1   2   3   4
Number of errors ....(14,15) ☐ ☐
Within normal limits Normal/3 pts below/4 points/5 or more below   (16) ☐
                          1   2   3   4

Types of Errors and Number
  (i) *Omissions* 0,1,2,.... .9+   (17) ☐   (ii) *Distortions* 0, 1, . 9+   (18) ☐
(iii) *Perseverations* 0,1, .. .9+   (19) ☐   (iv) *Rotations* 0,1, . . .9+   (20) ☐
  (v) *Misplacements* 0,1, .. .9+   (21) ☐   (vi) *Size Errors* 0,1, . .9+   (22) ☐

13. *Finger Sense*
                                            10%   5%
One or two fingers No. of errors RH .... Normal/Abnormal/Critical (23) ☐
                                              1   2   3
                          LH .... Normal/Abnormal/Critical (24) ☐
                                              1   2   3
In-between fingers No. of errors RH .... Normal/Abnormal/Critical (25) ☐
                                              1   2   3
                          LH .... Normal/Abnormal/Critical (26) ☐
                                              1   2   3

14. *Problems of Position*

Part I. Score .....(27,28) ☐ ☐   Part II. Score .... (29,30) ☐ ☐

Number of errors   1. Mirror Image (31) ☐   2. Inverted   (32) ☐

3. Inversion 180′ (33) ☐ 4. Clockwise 90′(34) ☐   5. Anti-   (35) ☐

Stott

W—withdrawal	(36) ☐	U—unforthcomingness	(37) ☐
D—depression	(38) ☐	XA—anxiety to adults	(39) ☐
HA—hostility to adults	(40) ☐	K—indifference to adults	(41) ☐
XC—anxiety to children	(42) ☐	HC—hostility to children	(43) ☐
R—restlessness	(44) ☐	(M—emotional tension	(45) ☐)
Total (excl.M,MN)	(47,48) ☐ ☐	(MN—Nervousness	(46) ☐)

Confidential   BG—1

BRISTOL SOCIAL-ADJUSTMENT GUIDES—No. 1

THE CHILD IN SCHOOL—(BOY)

(For the Observation of Day-School Children, 5-15 years).

Prepared by D. H. Stott, Ph.D. and Miss E. G. Sykes

The object of this Guide is to give a picture of the child's behaviour and to help in the detection of emotional instability.

Name of child..

Birth date.............. Date of this record..................

Teacher making record.......................................

School ....

METHOD OF USE

Underline in ink the phrases which describe the child's behaviour or attitudes over the past term or so. If any feature is very marked, underline twice. More than one item may be underlined in each paragraph, but do not underline any unless definitely true of the child. Add any remarks necessary beside the underlining, or at the end of the Guide. Where an item seems inappropriate because of age, etc., it can be ignored. If nothing is applicable mark 'n.n.' (nothing noticeable). Do not bother to *rule* underlinings.

ATTITUDES TOWARDS THE TEACHER

Greeting teacher:
Over-eager to greet/greets normally/sometimes eager sometimes definitely avoids/ waits to be noticed before greeting/absolutely never greets/n.n.

Response to greeting:
Usually friendly/can be surly or suspicious/mumbles shyly, awkwardly/does not answer/answers politely/n.n.

Helping teacher with jobs:
Always willing/very anxious to do jobs/offers except when in a bad mood/ never offers but pleased if asked/has no wish to volunteer/n.n.

Answering questions:
Always ready to answer/sometimes eager sometimes doesn't bother/eager except when in one of his moods/gets nervous, blushes, cries when questioned/not shy but unconcerned/n.n.

Asking teacher's help:
Always finding excuses for engaging teacher/seeks help only when necessary; seldom needs help/too shy to ask/not shy but never comes for help willingly/ too apathetic to bother/at times very forward, at times unsociable/depends on how he feels.

General manner with teacher:
Natural, smiles readily/over-friendly/shy but would like to be friendly/makes no friendly or eager response/sometimes friendly, sometimes in a bad mood/ quite cut off from people, you can't get near him as a person/not open or friendly; sometimes 'seems to be watching you to see if you know'/n.n.

Talking with teacher:
Normally talkative/forward (opens conversation)/over-talkative (tires with constant chatter)/inclined to be moody/says very little; can't get a word out of him/ avoids talking (distant, deep)/avoids teacher but talks to other children.

Talks to t. about own doings, family or possessions—normally for age/excessively/ never makes any first approach/chats only when alone with teacher/n.n.

Contacts with teacher:
Very anxious to bring/sometimes brings/never brings flowers, gifts, although classmates often do.

Brings objects he has found, drawings, models, etc. to show teacher—very often/ sometimes/never, although classmates often do.

Sidles up to or hangs round teacher/minimises contacts but not backward with other children/like a suspicious animal/n.n.

Liking for attention:
Appreciates praise/tries to monopolise t./put out if he can't get attention/ wants adult interest but can't put himself forward/suspicious (on the defensive)/ unconcerned about approval or disapproval.

Liking for sympathy:	Craves for sympathy (comes unnecessarily with minor scratches, bumps, etc., complains of being hurt by others)/doesn't make unnecessary fuss/keeps clear of adults even when hurt or wronged/likes sympathy but reluctant to ask/takes advantage of sympathy or interest/n.n.
Classroom behaviour:	Well-behaved/too timid to be naughty/occasionally naughty/has no life in him/ constantly needs petty correction/very naughty, difficult to discipline/plausible, sly; will abuse trust, hard to catch/n.n.
Truthfulness:	Always or nearly always truthful/lies from timidity/sometimes a fluent liar/ habitual slick liar; has no compunction about lying/tells fantastic tales.
Honesty:	Copies from others/normally honest with school work.
	'Borrows' books from desks without permission/has stolen money, sweets (candy), valued objects—frequently/once or twice/never.
Attitude to correction:	Normal for age/bursts into tears/resentful muttering or expression at times/ aggressive defiance (screams, threats, violence)/plays the hero.
Effect of correction:	Behaves better/too immature to heed/too restless to remember for long/can't resist playing to the crowd/bears a grudge, always regards punishment as unfair/ becomes antagonistic/treats lenience as weakness/n.n.

ATTITUDE TO SCHOOL WORK

Attentiveness:	Apathetic ('just sits')/won't bother to learn/dreamy and distracted ('lives in another world')/cannot attend or concentrate for long (cannot sit still when read to or during broadcasts, plays with things under desk, etc.)/n.n.
Persistence (classwork):	Works steadily/too restless ever to work alone/works only when watched or com-pelled/can work alone but has no energy/varies very noticeably from day to day.
Classwork standard:	Reading (English): Good/average/poor for age/cannot read. Arithmetic (Math): Good/average/poor for age/completely incompetent.
Persistence (manual tasks):	Sticks to job/gives up easily/impatient, loses temper with job/depends on his mood/varies greatly/lacks physical energy/works only when watched or com-pelled/distant and uninterested.
Standard (manual):	Work good or average/very erratic (seems at times to do badly on purpose)/ rough-and-ready, slapdash.

GAMES AND PLAY

Team games:	Plays steadily and keenly; with great energy/eager to play but loses interest/ inclined to fool around/dreamy, uninterested/always sluggish, lethargic/ sometimes alert, sometimes lethargic/n.n.
	Fits in well with team/bad loser (makes a fuss when game goes against him)/ bad sportsman (plays for himself only, cheats, fouls)/submissive, takes less wanted position, a 'ball fetcher'.
	Over-brave (takes unnecessary risks)/timid, poor-spirited; can't let himself go/ normally courageous.
Informal play:	Shrinks from active play/plays childish games for his age/healthily noisy and boisterous/starts off others in scrapping and rough play/disturbs others' games; teases, likes to frighten others/n.n.
Individual games:	Likes sedentary games (board games, cards, etc.)/is too restless/good loser/bad loser. Honest/cunning, dishonest/n.n.
Free activity:	Can always amuse himself; works patiently at models, etc./does not know what to do with himself, can never stick at anything long/sometimes lacks interest/n.n.

Favourite activity ....

ATTITUDES TO OTHER CHILDREN

Companionship: Good mixer/associates with one other child only and mostly ignores the rest/ distant, shuns others/sometimes wanders off alone/can never keep a friend long (tries to pal up with newcomers)/over-anxious to be in with the gang (tries to buy favour with others, easily led)/likes to be the centre of attention/mostly on bad terms with others.

Ways with other children: Gets on well with others; generally kind, helpful/sometimes nasty to those outside own set/squabbles, makes insulting remarks/selfish, scheming, a spoil sport/ hurts by pushing about, hitting/spiteful to weaker children/tells on others, underhand (tries to get others into trouble)/n.n.

Plays only or mainly with older/younger children/those of own age.

Physical prowess: Never fights/fights gamely/gets bullied/strikes brave attitudes but backs out/ flies into a temper if provoked/fights viciously (bites, kicks, scratches, uses dangerous objects as weapons)/n.n.

Liking the limelight: Brags to other children. Shows off (makes silly faces, mimics, clowns). Misbehaves when teacher is out of room/n.n.

Attitude of other children: Liked/disliked, shunned/on the fringe, somewhat of an outsider/associates mostly with unsettled types/gets cheated, fooled.

PERSONAL WAYS

Attendance: Good/frequently absent for day or half-day/has had long absences/has truanted— once or twice, often, suspected of truancy/parent condones absences, malingering, etc./stays away to help parent.

Punctuality: Good or fairly good/often late/has cut lessons.

Belongings: Looks after books, etc./careless, untidy; often loses or forgets books, pen/ destructive, defaces with scribbling.

Ability at class jobs: Sensible/irresponsible, scatterbrain/untrustworthy/varies with mood/just stupid/n.n.

Care for appearance: Adopts extreme youth fashions/not much concerned with looks/slovenly, very dirty/ gets very dirty during day/smart and tidy for age/n.n.

Speech: Stutters, stammers, can't get the words out/thick, mumbling, inaudible/jumbled/ incoherent rambling chatter/babyish (mispronounces simple words)/n.n.

Eyes: Dull, listless/unresponsive (doesn't seem to see you)/can't look you in the face/ has a wild hostile look; looks from under brows/blinking/bright/n.n.

Posture: Slumps, lolls about/walks alertly/shuffles listlessly/n.n.

Expression: Miserable, depressed ('under the weather'), seldom smiles/vacant/serious/placid, complacent/perky/n.n.

Fidgets, etc.: Unwilled twitches, jerks; makes aimless movements with hands/bites nails badly. Jumpy/sucks thumb or finger (over ten years)/continually giggling/n.n.

Nuisance: Damage to public property, etc. (of school, fences, unoccupied houses)/damage to personal property (cars, delivery vehicles, occupied houses or gardens, teacher's or workmen's belongings, etc.)/foolish pranks when with a gang/spoils or hides other children's things/follower in mischief/bad language; vulgar stories, rhymes, drawings/obscene behaviour/n.n.

Sexual development: Early; very keen on opposite sex/normal/abnormal tendency/delayed.

Appearance: Attractive/not so attractive as most/looks undernourished/has some abnormal feature/n.n.

PHYSIQUE

General health: Poor breathing, wheezy, asthmatic, easily winded/frequent colds, tonsillitis, coughs; running nose; mouth breather/running, infected ears/skin troubles, sores/ complains of tummy aches, feeling ill or sick; is sometimes sick/headaches; bad turns, goes very pale; fits/nose-bleeding/sore, red eyes/very cold hands/ good health.

Physical defects: Bad eyesight; squint; bulging eyes; poor hearing; gawky (bad co-ordination); contorted features (face screwed up on one side, eyes half closed, etc.); holds limb or body in unnatural posture.

Size: Tall for age/ordinary/small/unusually small.   Very fat/very thin/n.n.

Anything special about this child which is not covered in the form.:

Summary, recommendations; comments:

SBN 340 06174 X

Eighth impression 1968
Copyright © 1956 D. H. Stott and E. G. Sykes.
All rights reserved. No part of this publication
may be reproduced or transmitted in any form or
by any means, electronic or mechanical, including
photocopy, recording, or any information storage
and retrieval system, without permission in
writing from the publisher.
University of London Press Ltd
St Paul's House, Warwick Lane, London EC4

Printed in Great Britain by
Chigwell Press Ltd, Buckhurst Hill, Essex

Page 4

Confidential — On completion please return to the Word Blind Centre, ICAA.

REPORT FROM SCHOOL

Date . . . .

Name of Child . . . . Sex . . . .

Date of Birth . . . . Age . . . . years . . . months . . .

Name of School . . . . Type . . . .

Address of School . . . .

. . . .

Date of Admission . . . . Class . . . .

School Work — Levels of attainments now

Reading . . . .

Spelling . . . .

Writing . . . .

English . . . .

Arithmetic . . . .

Drawing . . . .

Handwork . . . .

Music . . . .

Games, Sports . . . .

Gymnasium, PE . . . .

Swimming Ability . . . .

Other Subjects . . . .

Strongest Subject . . . .

Weakest Subject . . . .

Special Abilities and Interests . . . .

. . . .

Is this child attending a special class for backward children or receiving special attention? (Please give details) . . . .

. . . .

Behaviour

In Classroom . . . .

. . . .

In Playground . . . .

. . . .

Outside School . . . .

. . . .

At Home . . . .
(if known)

. . . .

Attitudes
To Teachers . . . .
. . . .
To older Children. . . . .
. . . .
To younger Children . . . .
. . . .
To others . . . .
. . . .
Is child member of any juvenile organization? If so which? . . . .
. . . .

School Difficulties (other than attainment)
Attendance. . . . .
Any others. . . . .

Parents
Are parents interested in child's progress? . . . .
. . . .
Interested in child's behaviour? . . . .
How is parental interest, or lack of it, shown to child, and/or school? . . . .
. . . .

Bodily Characteristics
Physique (compared with class mates) . . . .
. . . .
Defects, Ill health etc. . . . .
. . . .

Intelligence — estimated to be (tick one)
Very bright
Bright
Average
Below Average
Limited

Comments, if any. . . . .
. . . .
. . . .
. . . .

Information from School Records

(VB = very backward   W = weak   G = good   VG = very good)

Teachers estimates of quality of work	Infants	Years in Juniors				Years in Seniors			
		1	2	3	4	5	6	7	8
Reading									
Spelling									
Writing.									
English									
Arithmetic									
Drawing									
Handwork									
Other subjects									
No. of possible attendances .									
Actual attendances									
Position in Class									
No. of pupils in Class									
Average age of Class									

Information on Tests Performed
If the child has been given any tests by schools or clinics please supply details.

Name & Description of Tests used	*Date given*	*Results*
Psychological Tests		
. . . .	. . . .	. . . .
. . . .	. . . .	. . . .
Scholastic Tests		
Reading (Age)	. . . .	. . . .
Arithmetic (Age)	. . . .	. . . .
Others.	. . . .	. . . .
. . . .	. . . .	. . . .

Previous Psychological Treatment (if any)

Child Guidance?

Tutorial or remedial classes?

Individual coaching (school/home)?

Personality. Character Traits, etc.

It would be of immense help to us if the class teacher could check through the enclosed Bristol Social-Adjustment Guide. Please add any comments at the end of the form.

Additional Information

Please write here any comments or information which may be of value to us concerning this child.

Signature . . . .   Position in School . . . .

References

Altus, G. T. (1956) "A WISC profile for retarded readers." *Journal of Consulting Psychology*, **20**, p 155.

Asso, D., and Wyke, M. (1970) "Visual discrimination and verbal comprehension of spatial relations by young children." *British Journal of Psychology*, **61**, p 99

Bannatyne, A. D. (1966) "Diagnostic and remedial techniques for use with dyslexic children." *Word Blind Bulletin*, **1**, Nos 6 and 7.

Bax, M. C. O., and Mac Keith, R. (Eds.) (1963) "Minimal cerebral dysfunction." *Little Club Clinics in Developmental Medicine*, No 10.

Beery, J. W. (1967) "Matching of auditory and visual stimuli by average and retarded readers." *Child Development*, **38**, p 867.

Belmont, L., and Birch, H. G. (1965) "Lateral dominance, lateral awareness and reading disability." *Child Development*, **36**, p 57.

Belmont, L., and Birch, H. G. (1966) "The intellectual profile of retarded readers." *Perceptual and Motor Skills*, **22**, p 787.

Benton, A. L. (1958) "Significance of systematic reversals in left-right discrimination." *Acta Psychiatrica Neurologica*, **33**, p 129.

Benton, A. L. (1959) *Right-left Discrimination and Finger Localization*. New York, Hoeber.

Birch, H. G. (1962) "Dyslexia and the maturation of visual function," in *Reading Disability*, J. Money (Ed). Baltimore, Johns Hopkins Press.

Birch, H. G. (1964) *Brain Damage in Children*, H. G. Birch (Ed). Baltimore, Williams and Wilkins.

Birch, H. G., and Belmont, L. (1964) "Auditory-visual integration in normal and retarded readers." *American Journal of Orthopsychiatry*, **34**, p 852.

Birch, H. G., and Lefford, A. (1963) *Intersensory Development in Children*. Monograph of the Society for Research in Child Development, 89, 28, No. 5.

Boshes, B., and Myklebust, H. R. (1964) "A neurological and behavioural study of children with learning disorders." *Neurology*, **14**, p 7.

Brenner, M. W., and Gillman, S. (1966) "Visuomotor ability in schoolchildren – a survey." *Developmental Medicine and Child Neurology*, **8**, p 686.

Bruce, D. J. (1964) "The analysis of word sounds by young children." *British Journal of Educational Psychology*, **34**, p 158.

Burt, C. (1937) *The Backward Child.* University of London Press.
Burt, C. (1966) "Counterblast to dyslexia." *AEP News Letter,* No 5, p 2.
Chief Medical Officer of the Department of Education and Science (1969) "Children who have difficulty in learning," in *The Health of the School Child 1966—8.* HMSO
Clark, M. M. (1957) *Left-Handedness.* University of London Press.
Clark, M. M. (1970) *Reading Difficulties in Schools.* Penguin Papers in Education. Penguin Books.
Clarke, G. Lady Brenda (1966). Personal Communication.
Cohn, R. (1961). "Delayed acquisition of reading and writing abilities in children: a neurological study." *Archives of Neurology,* 4, p 153.
Collins, J. E. (1961) *The Effects of Remedial Education.* Educational Monograph IV, University of Birmingham Institute of Education.
Critchley, M. (1962) "Developmental dyslexia: a constitutional dyssymbolia" in *Word-blindness or Specific Developmental Dyslexia.* A. W. Franklin (Ed). London, Pitman Medical, p 45.
Critchley, M. (1964) *Developmental Dyslexia.* London, William Heinemann Medical Books Ltd. Now out of print — 2nd edition 1970, *The Dyslexic Child.*
Crosby, R. M. N., with Liston, R. A. (1968) *Reading and the Dyslexic Child.* London, Souvenir Press.
Daniels, J. C. (1962) "Reading difficulty and aural training," in *Word-blindness or Specific Developmental Dyslexia,* A. W. Franklin (Ed). London, Pitman Medical.
Davis, D. R., and Kent, N. (1955) "Intellectual development in school children with special reference to family background." *Proceedings of the Royal Society of Medicine,* 48, p 933.
Davis, E. A. (1937) *The Development of Linguistic Skills in Twins, Singletons with Siblings and only children from Age Five to Ten Years.* Minneapolis, University of Minnesota Press.
Debray, P. (1968) "La dyslexie de l'enfant." *Gazette Médicale de France,* 75, p 5181.
De Hirsch, K., Jansky, J. J., and Langford, W. S. (1966) *Predicting Reading Failure.* New York, Harper and Row.
De Séchelles, Mme. (1962) "The Treatment of Word-Blindness" (translation), in *Word-Blindness or Specific Developmental Dyslexia,* A. W. Franklin (Ed). London, Pitman Medical.
Doehring, D. G. (1968) *Patterns of Impairment in Specific Reading Disability.* Indiana University Press.
Eisenberg, L. (1962) *Introduction to Reading Disability,* Money, J. (Ed). Baltimore, Johns Hopkins Press.
Espir, M., and Russell, W. R. (1961) *Traumatic Aphasia.* London, Oxford University Press.
Ettlinger, G., and Jackson, C. V. (1955). "Organic factors in developmental dyslexia." *Proceedings of the Royal Society of Medicine,* 48, p 998.
Fildes, L. G. (1921) "A psychological inquiry into the nature of the condition known as congenital word-blindness." *Brain,* 44, p 286.
Fisher, J. H. (1905) "A case of congenital word-blindness (inability to learn to read)." *Oph. Rev.,* 24, p 315.
Fisher, J. H. (1910) "Congenital word-blindness (inability to learn to read)." *Trans. Oph. Soc. UK,* 30, p 216.

Francis-Williams, J. (1970) *Children with Specific Learning Difficulties.* Pergamon Press.

Franklin, A. W. (Ed) (1962) *Word-Blindness or Specific Developmental Dyslexia.* London, Pitman Medical.

Franklin, A. W. (1968) "A paediatrician looks at dyslexia." *Word Blind Bulletin,* 2, p 25.

Galifret-Granjon, N. (1952) "Le problème de l'organisation spatiale dans les dyslexics d'évolution," in *L'Apprentissage de la Lecture et ses Troubles.* Paris, Presses Universelles.

Galifret-Granjon, N. (1959) "L'élaboration des rapports spatiaux et la dominance latérale chez les enfants dyslexiques-dysorthographiques." *Bulletin de la Société Alfred Binet,* 6, p 452.

Galifret-Granjon, N., and **Ajuriaguerra, J.** de (1951) "Trouble de l'apprentissage de la lecture et dominance latérale." *Encéphale,* 3, p 385.

Gallagher, J. Roswell (1962) "Word-blindness (reading disability; dyslexia) its diagnosis and treatment," in *Word-Blindness or Specific Developmental Dyslexia,* A. W. Franklin (Ed). London, Pitman Medical.

Gates, A. I., and **Bond, G. L.** (1936) "Relation of handedness, eye-sighting and acuity dominance to reading." *Journal of Educational Psychology,* 27, p 450.

Gooddy, W. (1967) "The neurological aspects of dyslexia." Paper presented at a Seminar on Dyslexia sponsored by the Reading and District Hospital Management Committee, Reading County Borough Education and Health Committee, Royal County of Berkshire Education and Health Committees.

Gooddy, W., and **Reinhold, M.** (1961) "Congenital dyslexia and asymmetry of cerebral function." *Brain,* 84, p 231.

Gower, J. C., and **Ross, G. J. R.** (1969) "Minimum spanning trees and single linkage cluster analysis." *Applied Statistics,* 18, p 54.

Hallgren, B. (1950) "Specific Dyslexia." *Acta Psychiatrica Neurologica,* Supplement 65.

Harris, A. J. (1947) *How to Increase Reading Ability.* New York, Longmans Green.

Harris, A. J. (1957) "Lateral dominance, directional confusion and reading disability." *Journal of Psychology,* 44, p 283.

Harris, A. J. (1958) Harris Tests of Lateral Dominance. The Psychological Corporation, New York.

Hendrickson, L. N., and **Muehl, C.** (1962) "The effect of attention and motor response pre-training on learning to discriminate 'b' and 'd' in kindergarten children." *Journal of Educational Psychology,* 53, p 236.

Hermann, K. (1959) *Reading Disability.* Copenhagen, Munksgaard.

Hilman, H. H. (1956) "The effect of laterality on reading disability." *Durham Research Review,* 7, p 86.

Hinshelwood, J. (1895) "Word-blindness and visual memory." *Lancet,* 2, p 1564.

Hinshelwood, J. (1900) *Letter-, Word- and Mind-blindness.* London, Lewis.

Hinshelwood, J. (1917) *Congenital Word-blindness.* London, Lewis.

Holt, L. M. (1962) "The treatment of word-blind children at St. Bartholomew's," in *Word-Blindness or Specific Developmental Dyslexia,* A. W. Franklin (Ed). London, Pitman Medical.

Hood, J. D. (1970) Personal communication.

Humphrey, M. E., and **Zangwill, O. L.** (1952) "Dysphasia in left-handed patients with unilateral brain lesions." *Journal of Neurology, Neurosurgery and Psychiatry*, 15, p 184.

Ilg, F. L., and **Ames, L. B.** (1950) "Developmental trends in reading behaviour." *Journal of Genetic Psychology*, 76, p 291

Ingram, T. T. S. (1963) "The association of speech retardation and educational difficulties." *Proceedings of the Royal Society of Medicine*, 56, p 199.

Ingram, T. T. S. (1964) "The dyslexic child." *Word Blind Bulletin*, 1, No. 4, p 1

Ingram, T. T. S. (1969) "Developmental disorders of speech," in *Handbook of Clinical Neurology*. Vinken, P. J., and Brown, G. W. (Eds). Amsterdam, North Holland Publishing Co.

Ingram, T. T. S., and **Mason, A. W.** (1965) "Reading and writing difficulties in childhood." *British Medical Journal*, 5459, p 463.

Ingram, T. T. S., and **Reid, J. F.** (1956) "Developmental aphasia observed in a department of child psychiatry." *Archives of Diseases in Childhood*, 31, p 161

Inner London Education Authority (1969) *Literacy Survey – Interim Report.*

Johnson, D. J., and **Myklebust, H. R.** (1967) *Learning Disabilities; Educational Principles and Practice.* New York, Grune and Stratton.

Kahn, D., and **Birch, H. G.** (1968) "Development of auditory-visual integration and reading achievement." *Perceptual and Motor Skills*, 27, p 459.

Kawi, A. A., and **Pasamanick, B.** (1958) "Association of factors of pregnancy with reading disorders in childhood." *Journal of the American Medical Association*, 166, p 1420.

Kawi, A. A., and **Pasamanick, B.** (1959) *Prenatal and Paranatal Factors in the Development of Reading Disorders.* Monograph of the Society for Research in Child Development, 24, No 4.

Kerr, J. (1897) "School hygiene, in its mental, moral and physical aspects." *Journal of the Royal Statistical Society*, 60, p 613.

Kinsbourne, M., and **Warrington, E. K.** (1962) "A study of finger agnosia." *Brain*, 85, p 47.

Kinsbourne, M., and **Warrington, E. K.** (1963 *a*) "The development of finger differentiation." *Quarterly Journal of Experimental Psychology*, 15, p 132.

Kinsbourne, M., and **Warrington, E. K.** (1963 *b*) "Developmental factors in reading and writing backwardness. *British Journal of Psychology*, 54, p 145.

Krise, E. M. (1952) "An experimental investigation of the theories of reversals in reading." *Journal of Educational Psychology*, 43, p 408.

Lachmann, F. M. (1960) "Perceptual-motor development in children retarded in reading ability." *Journal of Consulting Psychology*, 24, p 427.

Leroy-Bussion, A., and **Dupessey, C.** (1969) "Apprentissage de la lecture et synthèse des sons du language: Aptitude à restructurer un message orale fragmenté en syllabes chez les enfants de 4 à 7 ans." *Enfance*, 3–4, p 183

Lovell, K., and **Gorton, A.** (1968) "A study of some differences between backward and normal readers of average intelligence." *British Journal of Educational Psychology*, 36, p 240.

Lovell, K., **Gray, E. A.**, and **Oliver, D. E.** (1964) "A further study of some cognitive and other disabilities in backward readers." *British Journal of Educational Psychology*, 34, 275.

Lovell, K., Shapton, D., and **Warren, N. S.** (1964) "A study of some cognitive and other disabilities in backward readers of average intelligence as assessed by a non-verbal test." *British Journal of Educational Psychology*, **34**, 58.

Lucas, A. R., Rodin, E. A., and **Simson, C. B.** (1965) "Neurological assessment of children with early school problems." *Developmental Medicine and Child Neurology*, 7, p 143.

Lyle, J. G. (1969) "Reading retardation and reversal tendency: a factorial study." *Child Development*, **40**, p 832.

Lyle, J. G. (1970) "Certain antenatal, perinatal and developmental variables and reading retardation in middle-class boys." *Child Development*, **41**, p 481.

Lyle, J. G., and **Goyen, J.** (1968) "Visual recognition, developmental lag and strephosymbolia in reading retardation." *Journal of Abnormal Psychology*, **73**, p 25.

Lyle, J. G., and **Goyen, J.** (1969) "Performance of retarded readers on the WISC and educational tests." *Journal of Abnormal Psychology*, **74**, p 105.

McLeod, J. (1969) *Handbook for Dyslexia Schedule and School Entrance Check List*. University of Queensland Press.

Macmeeken, M. (1939) *Ocular Dominance in Relation to Developmental Aphasia*. University of London Press.

Malmquist, E. (1958) *Factors related to reading disabilities in the first grade of elementary school*. Stockholm, Almquist and Wiksell.

Mason, A. W. (1967) "Specific (developmental) dyslexia." *Developmental Medicine and Child Neurology*, **9**, p 183.

Meredith, G. P. (1962) "Psycho-physical aspects of word-blindness and kindred disorders," in *Word-Blindness or Specific Developmental Dyslexia*. A. W. Franklin (Ed). London, Pitman Medical.

Miles, T. R. (1962) "A suggested method of treatment for specific dyslexia," in *Word-Blindness or Specific Developmental Dyslexia*, A. W. Franklin (Ed). London, Pitman Medical.

Miles, T. R. (1970) *On Helping the Dyslexic Child*. Education Paperbacks. London. Methuen Educational Ltd.

Milner, B. (1962) "Laterality effects in audition," in *Interhemispheric Relations and Cerebral Dominance*. Mouncastle, V. B. (Ed). Baltimore, Johns Hopkins Press.

Milner, B., Branch, C., and **Rasmussen, T.** (1964) "Observations on cerebral dominance," in *Disorders of Language*, A. V. S. de Reuck and M. O'Connor, (Eds). London, Ciba.

Mittler, P. (1969) "Genetic aspects of psycholinguistic abilities." *Journal of Child Psychology and Psychiatry*, **10**, p 165.

Money, J. (1962) "Dyslexia: A postconference review," in *Reading Disability*, J. Money (Ed). Baltimore, Johns Hopkins Press.

Monroe, M. (1932) *Children who Cannot Read*. University of Chicago Press.

Morgan, W. Pringle (1896) "A Case of Congenital Word-blindness." *British Medical Journal*, 2, p 1378.

Myklebust, H. R., and **Johnson, D. J.** (1962) "Dyslexia in children." *Exceptional Children*, **29**, p 14.

Naidoo, S. (1961) *An Investigation into Some Aspects of Ambiguous Handedness*. M. A. Thesis, University of London.

Nettleship, E. (1901) "Cases of congenital word-blindness (inability to learn to read)." *Ophthal. Rev.*, **20**, p 61.

Newton, M. (1970) "A neuro-psychological investigation into dyslexia," in *The Teaching and Assessment of Dyslexic Children*, A. W. Franklin, and S. Naidoo, (Eds). London, I.C.A.A.

Orton, S. T. (1925) "Word-blindness in school children." *Archives of Neurology and Psychiatry*, **14**, p 581.

Orton, S. T. (1928) "Specific reading disability — strephosymbolia." *Journal of the American Medical Association*, **90**, p 1095.

Orton, S. T. (1937) *Reading, Writing and Speech Problems in Children*. London, Chapman & Hall.

Penfield, W., and Roberts, L. (1959) *Speech and Brain Mechanisms*. Princeton University Press.

Piaget, J. (1928) *Judgment and Reasoning in the Child*. New York, Harcourt, Brace.

Prechtl, H. F. R. (1962) "Reading difficulties as a neurological problem in children," in *Reading Disability*, J. Money (Ed). Baltimore, Johns Hopkins Press.

Pringle, M. L. Kellmer (1965) *Deprivation and Education*. London, Longman.

Pringle, M. L., Kellmer, Butler, N., and Davie, R. (1966) *11,000 Seven-year-olds*. London, Longman.

Rabinovitch, R. D. (1968) "Reading problems in children: definitions and classifications," in *Dyslexia*, A. H. Keeney and V. T. Keeney, (Eds). Saint Louis, The C. V. Mosby Co.

Rabinovitch, R. D., Drew, A. L., De Jong, R. N., Ingram, W., Withey, L. (1954) "A research approach to reading retardation." *Research Publications of the Association for Research in Nervous and Mental Diseases*, **34**, p 363.

Ravènette, A. T. (1968) *Dimensions of Reading Difficulties*. London, Pergamon Press.

Registrar-General (1960) *Classification of Occupations*. HMSO.

Reid, W. R., and Schoer, L. (1966) "Reading achievement, social class and subtest pattern on the WISC." *Journal of Educational Research*, **59**, p 469.

Reinhold, M. (1962) "The diagnosis of congenital dyslexia," in *Word-Blindness or Specific Developmental Dyslexia*, A. W. Franklin, (Ed). London, Pitman Medical.

Riis-Vestergaard, I. (1962) "Treatment at the Word-Blind Institute, Copenhagen," in *Word-Blindness or Specific Developmental Dyslexia*, A. W. Franklin (Ed). London, Pitman Medical.

Rutherfurd, W. J. (1909) "The aetiology of congenital word-blindness with an example." *British Journal of Children's Diseases*, **6**, p 484.

Rutter, M. L., Tizard, J., and Whitmore, K. (Eds) (1970) *Education, Health and Behaviour*. London, Longman.

Schilder, P. (1944) "Congenital alexia and its relation to optic perception." *Journal of Genetic Psychology*, **65**, p 67.

Schonell, F. J. (1950) *Backwardness in the Basic Subjects*. Edinburgh, Oliver and Boyd.

Schonell, F. J. (1962) *The Psychology and Teaching of Reading*. Edinburgh, Oliver and Boyd.

Shankweiler, D. P. (1962) "Some critical issues concerning developmental dyslexia," in *Word-Blindness or Specific Developmental Dyslexia*, A. W. Franklin (Ed). London, Pitman Medical.

Shearer, E. (1968) "Physical skills and reading backwardness." *Educational Research*, **10**, p 197.

Shedd, C. L. (1968) "Dyslexia clinical management," *Journal of Learning Disabilities*, **1**, p 171.

Silver, A. A., and **Hagin, R. A.** (1960) "Specific reading disability: delineation of the syndrome and relationship to cerebral dominance." *Comprehensive Psychiatry*, **1**, p 126.

Silver, A. A., and **Hagin, R. A.** (1964) "Specific reading disability: follow-up studies." *American Journal of Orthopsychiatry*, **34**, p 95.

Smith, L. C. (1950) "A study of laterality characteristics of retarded readers and reading achievers." *Journal of Experimental Education*, **18**, p 321.

Stephenson, S. (1907) "Six cases of congenital word-blindness affecting three generations of one family." *The Ophthalmoscope*, **5**, p 482.

Stott, D. H. (1963) *The Social Adjustment of Children*, Manual to the British Social Adjustment Guides. University of London Press.

Stott, D. H. (1966) "A general test of motor impairment for children." *Developmental Medicine and Child Neurology*, **8**, p 523.

Strauss, A. A., and **Kephart, N. C.** (1955) *Psychopathology and Education of the Brain-Injured Child*, Vol 2. New York, Grune and Stratton.

Swanson, R., and **Benton, A. L.** (1955) "Some aspects of the genetic development of right-left discrimination." *Child Development*, **26**, p 123.

Templin, M. (1957) *Certain Language Skills in Children*. University of Minnesota Press.

Thomas, C. J. (1905) "Congenital word-blindness and its treatment." *Opthalmoscope*, **3**, p 380.

Tjossem, T., Hansen, T., and **Ripley, H.** (1962) "An investigation of reading difficulty in young children." *American Journal of Psychiatry*, **118**, p 1104.

Vernon, M. D. (1958) *Backwardness in Reading*. Cambridge University Press.

Vernon, M. D. (1961) "Dyslexia and remedial education." Paper presented at a meeting of the English Division of Professional Psychologists, Nottingham.

Vernon, M. D. (1962) "Specific dyslexia." *British Journal of Educational Psychology*, **32**, p 143.

Vernon, M. D. (1970) "Specific developmental dyslexia," in *The Assessment and Teaching of Dyslexic Children*. A. W. Franklin and S. Naidoo (Eds). London, ICAA.

Warrington, E. K. (1967) "The incidence of verbal disability associated with retardation reading." *Neuropsychologia*, **5**, p 175.

Wechsler, D. (1949) *Wechsler Intelligence Scale for Children (Manual)*. New York, The Psychological Corporation.

Wepman, J. M. (1958) *Auditory Discrimination Test* (Manual). Distributed by NFER.

Wepman, J. M. (1960) "Auditory discrimination, speech and hearing." *Elementary School Journal*, **60**, p 325.

Witty, P. A., and **Kopel, D.** (1936) "Sinistral and mixed manual-ocular behaviour in reading disability." *Journal of Educational Psychology*, **27**, p 119.

Worster-Drought, C. (1962) "Some personal observations on dyslexia," in *Word-Blindness or Specific Developmental Dyslexia*, A. W. Franklin (Ed). London, Pitman Medical.

Zangwill, O. L. (1960) *Cerebral Dominance and its Relation to Psychological Function*. Edinburgh, Oliver and Boyd.

Zangwill, O. L. (1962 *a*) Discussion in *Word-Blindness or Specific Developmental Dyslexia*. A. W. Franklin (Ed). London, Pitman Medical.
Zangwill, O. L. (1962 *b*) "Dyslexia in relation to cerebral dominance," in *Reading Disability*, J. Money (Ed). Baltimore, Johns Hopkins Press.

Index

161